The Paris Diet

The Paris Diet

THE EUROPEAN REVOLUTION
IN WEIGHT CONTROL

Paul Sachet, M.D.,
and
Brian L. G. Morgan, Ph.D.,
with Roberta Morgan

VILLARD BOOKS   NEW YORK   1990

Library of Congress Cataloging-in-Publication Data

Sachet, Paul.
The Paris diet: the European revolution in weight control/by
Paul Sachet and Brian L. G. Morgan with Roberta Morgan.
p.   cm.
ISBN 0-394-58216-0
1. Low-calorie diet.   I. Morgan, Brian L. G.
II. Morgan, Roberta.   III. Title.
RM222.2.S2   1990
613.2'5—dc20   89-43465

Manufactured in the United States of America

3   5   7   9   8   6   4   2

FIRST EDITION

Book design by Carole Lowenstein

To fine food, fine wine, fine romance, and
a fine figure: bon appétit!

Before starting any diet and/or exercise plan, you should first have a thorough physical examination. Show your doctor the diet and get his approval. You may have certain conditions or be taking medications that will necessitate some alteration in the menus or special nutrient supplements, or the diet may be inappropriate for you.

Under no condition should children follow a restricted caloric plan of this type. Overweight adolescents may be put on a diet, but only under a doctor's strict supervision. Diabetics, pregnant women, lactating mothers, and people with such chronic health problems as heart or lung conditions or who are taking certain drugs (such as those for hypertension, depression, or diabetes)—must not follow the diet without consulting their physicians.

Having said that, we should also stress that there's no reason why most people can't follow this safe and medically tested plan with their physician's approval.

A Note from Paris

Before we introduce the Paris Diet, allow me first to introduce myself. I am Dr. Paul Sachet, nutritional consultant at the world-famous Nutrition Department of the Bichat Hospital in Paris. I have lived in Paris all my life and have traveled widely throughout the world, especially in Europe and the United States.

My job at the hospital is taking care of people with nutritional disorders—including excess weight problems—and so I have always been interested in new ways of helping people lose weight easily and safely. My patients have very specific dieting needs: They want to lose weight and still be able to eat gourmet meals.

After all, France is the land of great food, true? Paris has the well-deserved reputation of being the gastronomic capital of the world. Not only does it have many superb restaurants, but its population is fascinated with food. We love to talk about food, to exchange recipes and names of fine restaurants, and to try our hand at preparing *petits plats*. Eating well is one of our favorite hobbies. The foods in our specialized shops and open-air markets are so tempting and beautifully displayed that I often see tourists taking snapshots of them, right along with our historical monuments. Parisians constantly eat in three-star restaurants or in little country *auberges* serving gourmet food. Even at home, many prepare exquisite dishes for their families each and every night.

Parisians have another interest, as well: fashion and style. French women of all ages want to be slim enough to slip into those form-fitting Yves Saint-Laurent and Chanel suits. French couples want to look trim in their clinging ski outfits as they whiz down the slopes during the *sports d'hiver*.

How can these two desires be reconciled? Can a population keep at the same time both its fashionable physique and its inborn love of luscious food?

Ten years ago, I came to the conclusion that eating well and remaining trim and healthy actually *go together*. This is the very foundation of the Paris Diet. It makes it possible for everyone to look chic as well as to eat chic. The Paris Diet has been used by people from many countries whose cuisines are not exactly known for their "slimming" properties: Greece, West Germany, Holland, England, Switzerland, Brazil, Morocco, Saudi Arabia, Lebanon. These patients have come to me and have been thrilled with the results. They continue to enjoy delicious food, while losing all the weight they want. Some had already tried everything, from crash diets to faddish "cures"—with no success. Either they lost no weight at all or the weight came back once they stopped the diet. They came to me for a "last chance diet," as they called it, and the Paris Diet gave them that chance. After following the whole program, they lost weight, kept it off, and never had to diet again. Plus, many ate more and better food than before.

For more than ten years now, the Nutrition Department of the Bichat Hospital, headed by Professor Marian Apfelbaum, has helped more than thirty thousand overweight patients lose weight for good. The Paris Diet evolved from the principles of the basic diet advocated at Bichat.

The Paris Diet is not just another diet book; rather it's a book of diets. It isn't one basic diet made for everyone but a diet tailored to a very important individual: *you*. By using a four-stage diet divided into different programs, the Paris Diet gives you the ability to select the plan suited to your own special needs. For example, are you a life-dieter—someone who diets constantly or who always eats too little but still can't lose weight? Are you a recent weight-gainer? Are you very overweight, or do you have just a few pounds to lose? Do you love to cook gourmet meals, or would you prefer a simple eating plan? Whichever type of weight problem you have and whichever way you want to lose it, there's a diet in this book designed especially for you.

Whatever your personal requirements, the fact remains that most people with a weight problem like to eat. That's fine with me! Remember what I said at the beginning? The French remain slim even though they have had a lifelong love affair with food. In fact, they remain slim because of this affair. When you enjoy every morsel of what you eat (as you will on the Paris Diet, especially if you try our special Chef's Diet), you don't feel the need to overeat or to snack between meals. Ten years of experience at the Bichat Hospital, plus my successes with more than two thousand patients in my private practice, have taught me that many people fail to lose weight because they get bored with monotonous, bland diets. No one will have this problem on the Paris Diet. You won't have any problem shopping for or preparing the food on this diet, either. All the meals are easy to prepare, and noncooks can follow a plan developed for their needs.

Although the recipes come straight to you from some of the greatest chefs in Paris, the entire diet has been adapted for Americans by Dr. Brian Morgan, world-renowned nutritionist formerly of Columbia University's Institute of Human Nutrition. I was thrilled to have hosted Dr. Morgan in Paris for a series of lectures on nutrition and eating disorders. This is where we first met two years ago and developed the idea of bringing the Paris Diet across the Atlantic. The whole project was then organized and written by Roberta Morgan, noted author of many books and newsletters on dieting and health-related fields.

As you can see, a great deal of expertise along with numerous experiences with patients have been used to bring you this delicious, easy program for losing weight and keeping it off—the Paris Diet. Now all you have to do is try it: You have nothing to lose but your excess pounds.

Bonne chance et bon appétit!

PAUL SACHET, M.D.
Paris

Acknowledgments

This book has been a team effort in every sense of the word. We would like to thank the following people for their belief in this project, for their support, and for their tremendous assistance:

Samuel Mitnick, our agent; Diane Reverand of Villard Books, our editor; Jean-Pierre Letellier and Christian Vercelli, our *chefs de cuisine,* for preparing most of the chef's recipes; Susan Sarao, for adapting the recipes; Betsy Brown, for working with us on the exercise program; Anne-Marie Berthier, R.D., our dietician; Gabriel Landau, for his excellent translations of the chef's recipes; Marianne Sinclair, for additional translations; Brigitte Millot, for her secretarial services; the mail and phone services for connecting us all; and all the people who have already enjoyed the program as well as those who are just about to take the journey.

Contents

PART ONE

❖

Introducing The Paris Diet

*W*elcome to the world of delicious, satisfying food! Does that sound like a strange way to open a diet book? Well, this diet is like none you've ever seen or tried. It makes some dramatic but accurate promises:

You'll lose all the weight you want.
You won't be hungry.
You'll be able to eat more food than before.
You'll eat better and more delicious meals than before.
You'll never have to diet again!

Welcome to the Paris Diet, the revolutionary but simple eating program that has swept through Europe. From housewives to princesses, from secretaries to captains of industry, thousands of people have been thrilled with the results of this diet. They can eat out, eat well, drink, and enjoy their food without fear of weight gain. And they all lose weight on this program—every one—without gaining a pound back once they start eating normally again. Even a slip or two here and there no longer does any damage. That extra piece of pastry or glass of champagne won't expand the waistline and bring back those dieting blues.

The Paris Diet is designed for everyone. Whether you want to lose a little bit of weight or a lot, whether you diet all the time or this is the first time, whether you exercise regularly or not at all—the plan is easily tailored to your exact needs. It's simple to follow and contains a lot of variety. There are different menus to suit your preferences, from the most basic eating plans that can be used anywhere to recipes for exquisite gourmet dishes from the finest chefs in Paris. It's your choice.

What makes this diet so different, so delicious, yet so effective? The secret lies in the way it alters and corrects your metabolic rate by using specific foods. Your body will work to help you lose weight instead of working against you, which is the problem with most other diets. You see, the body compensates for weight loss by slowing its processes down, making it harder and harder to burn off calories. Each time you go on another diet, the body slows down even more. That's why people who eat very little or who constantly diet can't lose a pound unless they starve themselves. The Paris Diet changes all that. It gets your body back into the right gear, takes off the weight, then raises your food intake gradually so that your metabolism has time to adjust.

The basis of the diet is a four-stage plan: The first stage, the Preparation Program, has been designed for people with one of the most common eating problems—life-dieting. These are the people who eat too little rather than too much, who constantly go on and off diets, or who habitually restrict their food intakes. The Preparation Program raises their food intakes in order to prime their bodies for the second stage, the Weight Loss Program. The third stage, the Adjustment Program, increases their food intakes gradually to "set" the new weight. Finally, the fourth stage, the Maintenance Program, presents a hearty, healthy eating plan that keeps the extra pounds off for good. People who are not life-dieters can also use the multi-stage plan, although they usually start at the second stage. Chapter 3 tells you exactly how to adapt the diet to your own special needs.

In addition to losing weight, your whole appearance will improve by following the Paris Diet. The foods it contains will help your skin look younger, smoother, and clearer, while giving new life, body, and shine to your hair. The Paris Diet is also one of the healthiest programs around. It can help people with high cholesterol, high blood pressure, diabetes, hip and joint problems, or heart and lung conditions. You'll not only look better, you'll feel better too.

Being overweight, defined as being 10 percent or more over your ideal weight,* is a more serious threat than you might think: It can increase your risk for getting cancer, heart disease, diabetes, high blood pressure, lung disorders, gout, and osteoarthritis. Your odds

---

* To find your ideal body weight, see Table 2 on page 26.

for survival are worse during surgery. Moreover, overweight people can suffer from discrimination in the job market. So for the sake of your appearance, your health, and your loved ones, follow the Paris Diet, lose the extra weight, and keep it off permanently.

No one has to tell you that Parisians love to eat. They could never follow a diet that was boring, rigid, or unimaginative. At the same time, one of the characteristics of French chic is being slim. French men and women want to look sleek and sensual and are anxious to lose any extra pounds when they appear. This program has been developed with all these things in mind. It also includes a simple, quick exercise plan to tone up, firm up, and strengthen every part of your body during each part of the diet. Even at the lowest calorie stage, where no strenuous exercise is permitted, we have designed special stretching and strengthening workouts that will give you a boost of energy and keep you in great shape.

You may be worried that you won't be able to find the food in this diet or to cook it right or that the meals will take too long to prepare. Ease your mind! Great food doesn't have to be complicated. The ingredients are simple to find, and the dishes can be fixed in no time. And if you don't want to try these gourmet delights, you can follow our easy summary plans, which include commonly used foods and meals you can put together in minutes or order at almost any restaurant.

The best feature of the Paris Diet is the way you can eat afterward, and for the rest of your life. Until now, you may have been semi-starving yourself or eating bland foods to maintain your weight. Or perhaps you've been living in a state of guilt, binging on forbidden foods, gaining weight, then feeling terrible. Those days are over. After following our program, you can maintain your new weight by eating hearty, well-balanced, and delicious meals and not gain a single ounce back.

You'll look better, feel stronger, and be much healthier. You'll be ready to light up the boulevards of Paris, to find more romance in your life, and to climb every one of the steps in the Eiffel Tower.

That's a great goal to keep in mind, and it's our promise to you.

P. S., B. L. G. M, and R. M.
Paris, London, Miami, and New York

CHAPTER 1

How the Paris Diet
Can Change Your Life

*A*re you sick of eating only salads and dry tuna, with no results? Do you dread getting on a scale or buying new clothes even though you barely eat a thing? Do you eat normally but steadily gain weight? Do diets seem pointless because you never lose a pound no matter how carefully you follow them?

Many of you are nodding your heads right now. We know. We've seen it enough in the hospital and in private practice. Most people who have a weight problem eat very little, or at the worst, eat normally. And most diets they try fail, either because the plans are boring or impossible to follow or because they're not adjusted to different people's metabolic needs.

That's why the Paris Diet has been so successful. It works for everyone, it's easy to follow, and it permanently ends the need to starve yourself just to maintain your weight. You can lose all you need to on this program, and by the time you reach the Maintenance Program, you will be able to eat a great deal of food without gaining a pound.

Best of all, after following this program, you will never have to diet again.

Much of what you'll eat on the diet—especially if you follow the Chef's Menu—is so delicious you won't even believe you're dieting. Your taste buds will be satisfied, and because of our unique combinations of foods, you won't feel hungry.

Thousands have been helped permanently by the Paris Diet. Their figures have gone back to normal, their health has improved, they've been able to stop smoking without gaining weight, and many can now enjoy good food for the first time in their lives. We are thrilled by the improvements this program has made in the lives of so many people with different eating problems, just as you will be thrilled by the changes it makes in your life.

In this chapter we've included case histories so you can see how the program worked for our patients. Perhaps you'll recognize your own problem among these stories and realize that you've found the solution at last. We will also explain the basis for the Paris Diet: a four-stage diet that lets you take weight off easily—and permanently —because it makes your body work for you, not against you.

The Life-Dieter

It's strange but true: One of the most common weight problems is caused by eating too little food, not too much. Many of the people we see complain that they nearly starve themselves but can't lose a pound. We call these people "life-dieters," and it is for them that the Paris Diet was originally designed. Life-dieting is just what it sounds like: always eating too little or always being on a diet. What occurs is that your body's processes are slowed to such a degree that you can't lose weight unless you literally eat nothing.

When Saudi Arabian Princess S., age fifty-five, came to the clinic in Paris for the first time, she had just returned from visiting her two sons, who were studying pre-law at Harvard. During the trip to Boston, she had gained five pounds, having previously gained eleven pounds during a three-week Mediterranean cruise on her yacht. Princess S. began to cry in the office when she learned of her sixteen-pound weight gain. She didn't understand what was happening to her. A few extra petits fours and one or two glasses of champagne a day couldn't have added this much weight. Yet the scales didn't lie.

We took an eating history and found out that after menopause she'd gained ten pounds within a year and decided to get the problem under control. When she wasn't traveling abroad (either alone or with her husband on affairs of state), she would eat almost nothing —too much of nothing, as it turned out. She would have only a cup of coffee for breakfast, then take the very lightest of lunches: usually a few green vegetables and some fruit. In this way she was able to keep her figure trim for three quarters of the year. The moment she went on a trip or cruise, her weight would shoot up. When she returned, she would again cut down her food intake, but it was getting harder to lose the extra weight. Now she rarely managed to shed more than one or two pounds, even though she might have gained five to ten. Princess S was getting thicker and thicker around the middle, while all her friends were swearing that she hardly ate anything at all.

In fact, she did eat very little—fewer than 1,000 calories a day—and that was her whole problem. Her body had grown accustomed to using less energy for its basic needs. The body tends to do that as protection, an adaptation from the days of famines and lean harvests. Instead of burning up 1,500 calories for daily chores and functions, the body slows down its metabolic rate so that only 1,000 calories are needed. Of course, this is disastrous when you're trying to lose weight. The problem becomes even worse when you overeat again, even for a short time. Because the body now needs only 1,000 calories to maintain weight, any energy taken in over that is stored as fat.

How the Paris Diet Worked for a Life-Dieter

The full Paris Diet—Preparation, Weight Loss, Adjustment, and Maintenance—is made for people (usually women) with a life-dieting problem. If you eat too little or have recently been dieting, this is the plan for you.

I. The Preparation Program (1,200–1,400 Calories)

The Preparation Program, on which the princess started, requires that you eat more than you normally do. This gets your body back into the right metabolic gear and primes it for weight loss. Because these carefully balanced meals are high in protein, you don't gain any extra weight.

Princess S. had been on a diet for more than three years. She agreed to follow the Preparation Program of first 1,200 and then 1,400 calories for two months, the optimum periods needed to read-just the metabolic rate of the body. For most people, one month is fine.

The princess managed to lose three pounds during this stage, even though she was following the Chef's Menu of gourmet dishes and eating better than she normally did. You, too, may lose weight during this part of the program, although you'll be eating more than before. Why does this happen? First of all, you may have been consuming small meals of high calorie foods that were not well balanced. The problem is sometimes *what* you eat, not how much. By using foods high in protein, the first stage of the diet aids weight loss since the body burns up more calories of protein than any other type of food. Also, by carefully balancing the diet and making sure that you eat three regular meals each day, your body doesn't crave snack foods (the downfall of the weight-conscious). A healthy breakfast and lunch will help you avoid cake and cookies at work; a satisfying dinner will end that munching late at night.

II. The Weight Loss Program (600–900 Calories)

The Weight Loss Program is where you see the pounds fall off quickly. After having eaten a normal amount for perhaps the first time in years during the Preparation Program, you switch to a low-calorie diet that is finally effective. Even though this diet is restricted, the food is still satisfying. Because of its high protein content, you won't feel hungry. If you follow the Chef's Menus, the meals you'll eat will amaze you.

Within three weeks of starting the Weight Loss Program, Princess S. lost eighteen pounds. She was now down to her ideal weight, but in order to maintain it without ever again having to diet, she proceeded, as all life-dieters must, to the Adjustment phase.

III. The Adjustment Program (1,200–1,400 Calories)

This stage uses the same foods and menus you followed for the Preparation Program, but here they are used to adjust your body back to a higher caloric intake without any weight gain. You may even lose a little more during this phase—Princess S. shed another two pounds.

IV. The Maintenance Program (1,600–2,000 Calories)

The Maintenance Program gradually increases your food intake in two stages (or three stages, if appropriate) to avoid weight gain. Eventually you'll reach a Maintenance plan you can use for the rest of your life. Some people have been dieting for so long that they must stay at 1,600 calories in order not to gain weight again, but most will be able to eat 1,800 or even 2,000 calories without putting on an extra ounce. When you consider the fact that many life-dieters have been eating 1,000 calories or less for years, you can see how this new eating program becomes a treat. It is the gold at the end of the rainbow—the extra bonus you'll get from losing weight the Paris Diet way. Not only will you be slimmer, but you'll also be able to eat big, delicious meals.

We promised you at the beginning that the Paris Diet was designed for all types of weight problems. So what if you're not a life-dieter? Perhaps you eat normally and have a weight problem. Maybe you eat a lot. Will the program work for you? Of course. That's the beauty of its design. It can be adapted for everyone. Chapter 3 clearly tells you which program will suit your own needs. For now, read on about our patients, and see how the Paris Diet works for different types of people.

The Chronic Eater

When Martine H. came to see us, she was depressed and desperate. The mother of four children, she complained that she had been overweight since her teens. During the course of her pregnancies, she had put on another forty pounds. She was thirty-two years old, weighed almost 170 pounds, and stood only five feet three inches tall.

Martine had tried everything, from diuretics to appetite suppressants to every diet on the market. The weight often came off, but whenever she stopped the particular treatment she gained everything back. By the time she came to our clinic, she was fed up. She didn't really believe the Paris Diet would work, but she wanted to try it as a last resort. "If this doesn't do it," she sighed, "I'll have to have my mouth wired shut."

Martine's eating habits were no joy, either. Most of the time she restricted herself to bland, tasteless foods so that she wouldn't be tempted to eat too much. The minute she gave in and had even one piece of cake, she gained again. She couldn't eat well, and yet she couldn't lose any weight. She felt trapped.

How the Paris Diet Worked for a Chronic Eater

The Paris Diet turned out to be Martine's answer. Because she was an average eater, not a life-dieter, she followed the program in the way best suited to her needs. If you eat between 1,500 and 2,400 calories per day, this will be your plan, too.

II. The Weight Loss Program

Normal or average eaters don't have to prepare their bodies to lose weight the same way that life-dieters do. They can skip the Preparation Program and go right to the Weight Loss Program, where they'll swiftly start to lose weight.

Martine followed the Weight Loss Program for a month. She was surprised by how tasty and unique the food was, and she was over-joyed to see that she had lost twenty-five pounds.

III. The Adjustment Program

Normal eaters also must increase their food intake gradually in order not to gain the weight back. Martine lost another nine pounds during this phase of the diet.

IV. The Maintenance Program

By slowly increasing her caloric intake, Martine was delighted to find that she could eat 1,800–2,000 calories a day without gaining weight, far more than she ate before. She could even have healthy snacks with her children when they came home from school.

Her total weight loss on the diet was thirty-five pounds. However, she needed to lose about twenty pounds more, so she stayed at 2,000 calories for two months (to make sure her new weight was "set"), then followed the three programs over again. The second time around, people tend to lose about two thirds of what they did initially because of the body's metabolic adjustments. Martine was no excep-tion. Her second time through yielded a twenty-three pound loss, and a very happy woman.

The Sudden-Gainer

Dominique B. was a thirty-three-year-old new mother. For the last five years, she had worked as a secretary for a pharmaceutical company in Geneva. She is tall, standing five feet seven inches in her bare feet. Her constant weight of 132 pounds suited her well. At the health club where she worked out with weights twice a week, no one believed that she'd just had a baby.

Dominique loved her job, her family, her friends, and her coworkers. But one day things changed. Her boss (who was more like a friend) and many of the people in her department were transferred to another lab, in Paris. The new department head was unfriendly, authoritative, and sometimes downright rude. The people he hired were aggressive and competitive. Dominique began to hate going to work. At the same time, her husband was sent to London by his company for two months.

Until this time, Dominique had been very careful about what she ate. Now, however, she started to snack on cookies and candy to ease her nerves at work. As soon as she got home, she would rush to the refrigerator and eat a chunk of cheese, sometimes even a second piece with bread and butter, and then prepare a big dinner for herself. After she put the baby to bed, she'd sit in front of the television for hours, running back and forth from the kitchen to the living room, getting snack after fattening snack. Chocolates and pastries were her favorites, and she sometimes ate enough to make her sick. She often felt bloated and tired and eventually stopped going to the gym.

By the time her husband returned home, her appearance had changed drastically. She had put on almost twenty pounds! Noting her husband's displeasure, along with her own discomfort, she came to see us. She knew that her eating habits had gotten out of control and that she was snacking on too many sweets. In fact, she was eating double the number of calories she ate before (and that was a lot of food; previously, Dominique had been a healthy eater with a daily intake of around 2,000 calories).

How the Paris Diet Worked for a Sudden-Gainer

Since Dominique wasn't a life-dieter, we started her on the same program as Martine.

II. The Weight Loss Program

From the moment she began the diet, Dominique felt and looked better. Best of all, because of the types of foods she was eating, she wasn't as hungry as before. She no longer had the urge to nibble at work, and when she got home, she didn't miss the chocolates in front of the television. Her lunch, which used to be too light, was now a proper meal with the right amount of protein, and it kept her satisfied throughout the day.

Three weeks later, Dominique had lost eleven pounds without feeling even one hunger pang!

III. The Adjustment Program

After two weeks on this stage, she had lost another nine pounds and regained her perfect figure. Instead of returning to the gym, she also started our exercise plan and began to tighten her body using our walk-jog program.

IV. The Maintenance Program

On this stage, Dominique was soon eating like everyone else and could even occasionally accept a few homemade cookies at work with no weight gain (after eating a proper Paris Diet lunch, that is).

Dominique's husband is now thrilled with her weight as well as with the new meals she learned from following the program. Their family doctor has commented that he's never seen either of them in better shape. Oh, and by the way, Dominique has a new job—modeling clothes for a local fashion magazine.

The Smoker

Dominique is an example of one type of person who has been helped enormously by the Paris Diet: someone who gains weight because of sudden overeating. The cause could be a new baby, a divorce, a relocation, or just overindulgence in high-calorie foods. Smokers who quit also fall into this category. Many people who give up an addiction to such substances as tobacco or alcohol substitute food for their old habits. When a person stops smoking, the metabolism slows down to some degree since nicotine is a powerful stimulant. This can cause a weight gain of as much as fifteen pounds even if the food intake remains exactly the same! Because of this weight gain, some continue to risk their lives and don't stop.

If a person follows the Paris Diet when he or she quits, not only will no weight be gained, but some may be lost, too.

Marc G. is a successful Parisian television news anchorman, forty-seven years of age. He is very attractive and enjoys the company of many beautiful women. He liked to smoke, drink, and overeat the wrong things, but he never seemed to put on weight. Two months before coming to see us he got the scare of his life. Overtired, overworked, and nervous, he felt a severe pain in his chest while in front of the camera. He began to sweat, had difficulty breathing, and felt a sharp pain shooting up his left arm and shoulder blade. He managed to get through the program but afterward went immediately to the hospital. He discovered that he'd suffered a mild heart attack.

Marc's doctor categorically ordered him to stop smoking (he was a two-pack-a-day man). Marc was worried. Quitting was bad enough, but he had several friends who had stopped abruptly and had put on large amounts of weight. Marc was a celebrity. He couldn't afford to change his appearance. He asked his cardiologist for advice and was referred to us.

We put his mind at ease. We told him that if he followed a few rules of better eating, he wouldn't gain any weight when he stopped smoking.

How the Paris Diet Worked for a Smoker

Heavier eaters (over 2,500 calories a day) who want to lose weight will usually start with the Adjustment Program, and then proceed to the Maintenance Program. Marc was a heavy eater, but he didn't need to lose weight, so he only had to follow one program.

IV. The Maintenance Program

We started Marc at 1,600 calories for a month. For lunch with his colleagues, he had a normal meal, consisting of such items as a tomato salad, fish with green beans, low-fat cheese, and a fruit salad. In the evenings he could enjoy more food, although for a time he had to stop going to restaurants and drinking the night away. He began to prepare for himself and his lady friends gourmet meals from the Chef's Menu. Marc couldn't believe it: He was eating what he liked, not smoking, and not gaining any weight. The only thing he missed was a drink at night, which he was allowed when he graduated to 1,800 calories. He also learned how to monitor his own eating habits. If he splurged the night before, he would for the next day or two eat meals from the Weight Loss Program.

Marc's heart episode happened two years ago. He is still not smoking, and his audience hasn't noticed any change in his appearance.

The Medicine Reactor

Joseph R., originally from Italy, suddenly found himself jobless at age thirty-seven when the American company he worked for closed down its Brussels office. He had an excellent résumé and impeccable references, but finding another position turned out to be difficult. He began to lose faith in himself. After talking about suicide, he was convinced by his wife to seek psychiatric help.

Joseph was put on a few different types of tranquilizers and antidepressants. Within a month, he had gained fifteen pounds and felt even worse about himself. The medication had increased his appetite and perhaps slowed his metabolism, so the gain was inevitable. After hearing about our program from a talk show on television, he came to the hospital to see us.

How the Paris Diet Worked for a Medicine Reactor

We knew at once that Joseph was depressed. We also understood that you can't give a desperate person a very strict diet because it might only serve to depress them further. Joseph was put on the following program:

II. The Weight Loss Program

Joseph was an average eater, so he started with this program, but because of his mood, we skipped the first stage (600 calories) and instead used only the second stage (900 calories) for two weeks. During this time he lost eleven pounds.

III. The Adjustment Program

Joseph followed this part of the diet for a month, and he lost another five pounds and went back to his normal weight. His wife prepared some of the meals from the Chef's Menu, and Joseph began to feel better.

IV. The Maintenance Program

Joseph used the first stage of the Maintenance Program (1,600 calories) for the three months that he remained on medication and in therapy, and he never felt hungry. Meanwhile, his doctors helped him to believe in himself again. Soon he got a new and even better job and discontinued psychiatric treatment.

Just as certain medicines (such as amphetamines) can cause a noticeable drop in weight, others can cause a weight gain, often by increasing the patient's appetite. The medicine can't be stopped, but the person doesn't want to become obese, either. The Paris Diet has solved this problem for many people. It satisfies their increased appetites because of the food it contains, but it doesn't add lots of calories.

As you can see, the Paris Diet works for all types of people: those who want to lose weight, to maintain weight, or simply to eat well-balanced and healthier meals. Whichever type you are, there is a plan for you. Just refer to Chapter 3 for a detailed explanation of which program you should follow.

The Paris Diet Menu Plans

There is enormous variety in the Paris Diet. Within each program, you have your choice of three types of eating:

1. THE SUMMARY PLANS: These guidelines are for busy people who

don't have the time to prepare food for set menus. They can be used at home, at the office, or in restaurants. Simply eat the types of foods listed in the summary in the exact amounts indicated. We have provided equivalency tables to give you substitutions for the foods listed. For instance, if you don't want ½ cup of grapefruit juice, the tables provide a substitute.

2. THE STANDARD DIETS: These are set menus for each day, with easy-to-prepare meals. Some have recipes, others don't. You can also use substitutions here.

3. THE CHEF'S MENUS: These menus are the jewels in the crown, the gourmet side of life. Filled with recipes from the most noted chefs in Paris, you won't believe you're dieting when you try these dishes.

You can also mix and match plans, as long as you stay within the particular program. For example, you may grab something from the Summary Plan to the first stage of the Preparation Program on Monday, follow the Standard Plan on Friday, and cook something from the Chef's Menu on Saturday night.

The Paris Diet gives you this wide range of choices because we know that boredom leads to failure. And to complement the eating program, please use the exercises in Chapter 12 to firm, tone, and strengthen your body. All together, it's a complete make-over system for your looks, your health, and your life. It's also the last diet program you'll ever have to follow.

———————— ✦ ————————

CHAPTER 2

How to Make
Your Metabolism
Help You Lose Weight

*D*o you diet constantly but don't shed a pound? Frustrating, isn't it? No matter how much you deprive yourself of those goodies and snacks, your weight seems set at one point. Even if you manage to lose a little bit after weeks of strict dieting, you gain it all back as soon as you eat normally again. This is because your body is actually working against you—it is preventing you from losing the weight you want.

The Paris Diet is going to eliminate this problem forever. Through its carefully designed eating programs, your body will be trained to work for you when you're dieting so that your efforts will quickly show in your waistline. And best of all, by the end of the plan, you'll be able to eat a lot of food without gaining weight. That's because this diet makes your metabolism a friend, not an enemy.

Metabolism is a word that gets used a lot today, but most of the information you hear about it is inaccurate or half-true. Diets claim that they can "speed up your metabolism" or "change your metabolism." In reality, there's probably nothing wrong with your body's natural rhythm—you just have to know how to keep it finely tuned. If you eat the wrong things or follow the wrong diet, you could find yourself with extra weight that your body won't let you lose.

People often believe they're overweight because of a metabolic condition. Sometimes this is true, but more often it's not. They simply eat the wrong things and too much of them. People can also disturb their rhythms by eating too little, and we'll explain how this happens. First, let's find out exactly what your metabolism is and how you can make it work for you.

The Metabolic Angle

Metabolism is a broad term used to mean all the chemical reactions going on in your body that are responsible for burning calories. A calorie is simply a measure of energy. Your basal metabolism is the energy needed to keep your heart, lungs, brain, kidneys, and other organs, including your skin, fat, and muscle, functioning normally. This basic need accounts for about two thirds of the calories you eat. The rest are used to move your body around.

Of course, we all don't have the same energy needs. The larger you are, for example, the greater your requirements. Someone who is six feet tall needs more energy than someone who is five feet. The amount of muscle versus fat is also important; the more muscle, the greater the need for energy because muscle requires more fuel to work than does fat. One reason why men need to eat more than women is that they have more muscle tissue.

The more exercise you get, the greater your energy output and daily needs will be. We should point out that it takes a lot of work to burn off weight through exercise alone. Table 1 gives you a good illustration of this.

In order for you to lose one pound of fat, you need to burn off 3,500 calories. This obviously requires a lot of time to achieve by just working out. But exercise coupled with a sensible diet can help you lose weight, tone up your metabolism, and tighten any flabby areas. For this reason, we have designed a special exercise program to accompany the Paris Diet, described in Chapter 12.

Getting Your Energy the Right Way

Where does all the energy your body needs come from? Basically it comes from the carbohydrate, fat, and protein in your daily meals, which also should provide you with vitamins and minerals. You see, all sources of nutrients are not created equal. Some are much better for you than others.

Americans eat in a far from perfect way, although their dietary habits have been improving. Up until now, they've consumed too much sugar, too much salt, too many calories, too much fat, and not

TABLE 1

Calories Burned Through Various Forms of Exercise

ACTIVITY	CALORIES BURNED PER MINUTE WEIGHT	
	(115–150 lb)	(150–195 lb)
aerobic dancing	6–7	8–9
basketball	9–11	11–15
bicycling	5–6	7–8
golf	3–4	4–5
jogging (5 mph)	9–10	12–13
jogging (7 mph)	10–11	13–14
rowing machine	5–6	7–8
skiing (downhill)	8–9	10–12
swimming	5–6	7–10
tennis (doubles)	5–7	7–8
walking (2 mph)	2–3	3–4
walking (4 mph)	4–5	6–7

enough fiber. For the sake of your future health, you must change your bad habits. The Paris Diet is a great place to start.

How does one type of nutrient differ from the other?

Carbohydrate is the most readily available source of energy in our bodies. We take it in as starch and refined sugar and store for future use a certain amount in our muscles and liver in a form called *glycogen.* Between meals, your body uses its store of carbohydrate to maintain the supply of energy to the body's tissues. These stores are also drawn on during vigorous exercise. The brain has a constant need for carbohydrate and burns about 450 calories each day.

Unfortunately, only a small amount of carbohydrate can be stored as glycogen, and any excess we eat is turned into fat. Simple carbohydrate such as sugar contains calories (4 calories per gram, or 120 per ounce) but no other useful nutrients. Complex carbohydrate, on the other hand, contains the equivalent calories but is rich in nutrients that are essential to good health. You should avoid simple sugars as much as possible and incorporate complex carbohydrates into your daily diet. The following is a quick reference list of food sources for the two different types of carbohydrates.

Sources of Simple Versus Complex Carbohydrates

SIMPLE	COMPLEX
cakes	beans (any kind)
candies	breads
cookies	carrots
corn syrup	cereals (unsweetened, any kind)
fruit juice*	corn
honey	crackers
jams	nuts
jellies	parsnips
molassses	pasta
soda	peas
sugar, maple	potatoes
sugar, table	yams

* Fruit juices are an exception to the rule of simple versus complex carbohydrates because they are also rich in an essential nutrient—vitamin C.

Among the carbohydrates, you should also avoid such refined foods as white breads, cakes, processed breakfast cereals, cookies, and buns unless they are enriched. During refinement, vitamins and minerals are lost, and so whole-wheat products generally have a greater nutrient content and a higher level of fiber (essential for a healthy digestive tract).

Fats are the second supplier of energy in our diets. They contain the highest amount of calories: 9 per gram, or 270 per ounce. Fats come in three forms—saturated, monounsaturated, and polyunsaturated. In general, saturated fats increase blood cholesterol levels, while polyunsaturates, and to a lesser degree, monounsaturates, decrease cholesterol levels. However, there is a great deal of individual variation and not everyone will react to fats in this way. Nonetheless, it is best if you stick to a diet low in fat, such as the Paris Diet.

The following is a list of foods that are high or low in fat.

Low Versus High Fat Foods

LOW	HIGH
beef: bottom, top, ground, or eye round; sirloin tip; roast filet; rump; flank, minute, or cube steak	beef: shell strip; T-bone, club, sirloin, chuck, or porterhouse steak; filet mignon; rib or shoulder roast; short ribs; tongue
chicken, without skin	butter, margarine, and oil
Cornish hen, without skin	cold cuts
fish, all types	duck
lamb: roast leg, steaks	frankfurters
pork: lean cured ham, lean ham steak	goose
shellfish, all types	lamb: shanks, loin or rib chops, stew
turkey, without skin	pork: loin chops, roast loin, Canadian bacon, bacon, spare ribs, salt pork, ham hocks
veal, all cuts	
vegetables and fruit, all except avocados and coconuts	

Protein can also serve as a source of energy, although its main functions include building new tissues; making neurotransmitters (chemical messengers in the brain), hormones, and enzymes (substances that control every chemical reaction in your body); and transporting essential nutrients around the body via the blood. Protein yields 4 calories per gram, or 120 calories per ounce of energy, the same as carbohydrate. The following is a list of foods that are high in protein:

Protein-Rich Foods

FOOD	SERVING SIZE	PROTEIN (grams)
beans, baked	1 oz	13
beef, lean, cooked	3 oz	23
beef, ground, cooked	3 oz	22
beef, sirloin steak, lean or fat, cooked	3 oz	20
bluefish, cooked	3 oz	22
calf's liver, fried	3 oz	25
cheese, American	1 oz	6
cheese, Cheddar	1 oz	6
cheese, cottage, creamed	1 cup	28
cheese, cottage, low fat (2%)	1 cup	31
cheese, Swiss	1 oz	8
chicken breast, cooked	3 oz	28
chicken drumstick, boned, cooked	3 oz	28
clams, raw	3 oz	11
egg	1	6
halibut, cooked	3 oz	21
ice cream	½ cup	3
ice milk	½ cup	3.2
lamb chop, cooked	3 oz	18
lentils, cooked	1 cup	16
lima beans, cooked	1 cup	16
milk, low fat (2%)	1 cup	8
milk, whole	1 cup	8
oatmeal, cooked	1 cup	5
peanuts, roasted	1 oz	8
pork, loin, cooked	3 oz	21
salmon, cooked	3 oz	17
shrimp, cooked	3 oz	21
sunflower seeds	1 oz	7
tuna, water packed	3 oz	24
turkey, dark, cooked	3 oz	26
turkey, white, cooked	3 oz	28
veal cutlet, cooked	3 oz	23
yogurt, low fat, plain	1 cup	9

Of these three energy sources, protein is the best to consume in a weight loss program because the body uses it less efficiently than either carbohydrate or fat. Why is less efficient better? For every 100 calories you take in as protein, only 80 can be used by the body. The rest is burned off as heat. With carbohydrate and fat, the body uses 90 calories for every 100 you take in. The more used, the more stored, the more turned into fat. In other words, a high-protein diet lets you eat a greater amount of food for fewer calories. That's why the Paris Diet uses so many protein-rich foods.

Maintaining the Right Weight

This book will show you how to get down to your ideal weight. But how do you find out what is ideal? First, measure your frame size. Place a tape measure around your wrist, right below your hand where the two bones on either side jut out. Then check this table:

HEIGHT WITHOUT SHOES	WRIST CIRCUMFERENCE	FRAME SIZE
4′8″ to 5′ 2″	< 5½″	small
	5½″ to 5¾″	medium
	> 5¾″	large
5′2″ to 5′5″	< 6″	small
	6″ to 6¼″	medium
	> 6¼″	large
> 5′5″	< 6¼″	small
	6¼″ to 6½″	medium
	> 6½″	large

Now, refer to Table 2 and see what your ideal weight is for your height.

TABLE 2
Ideal Weights According to Gender, Frame Size, and Height

MEN				
HEIGHT		SMALL	MEDIUM	LARGE
FEET	INCHES	FRAME	FRAME	FRAME
5	2	128–134	131–141	138–150
5	3	130–136	133–143	140–153
5	4	132–138	135–145	142–156
5	5	134–140	137–148	144–160
5	6	136–142	139–151	146–164
5	7	138–145	142–154	149–168
5	8	140–148	145–157	152–172
5	9	142–151	148–160	155–176
5	10	144–154	151–163	158–180
5	11	146–157	154–166	161–184
6	0	149–160	157–170	164–188
6	1	152–164	160–174	168–192
6	2	155–168	164–178	172–197
6	3	158–172	167–182	176–202
6	4	162–176	171–187	181–207

WOMEN				
HEIGHT		SMALL	MEDIUM	LARGE
FEET	INCHES	FRAME	FRAME	FRAME
4	10	102–111	109–121	118–131
4	11	103–113	111–123	120–134
5	0	104–115	113–126	122–137
5	1	106–118	115–129	125–140
5	2	108–121	118–132	128–143
5	3	111–124	121–135	131–147
5	4	114–127	124–138	134–151
5	5	117–130	127–141	137–155
5	6	120–133	130–144	140–159
5	7	123–136	133–147	143–163
5	8	126–139	136–150	146–167
5	9	129–142	139–153	149–170
5	10	132–145	142–156	152–173
5	11	135–148	145–159	155–176
6	0	138–151	148–162	158–179

Note: The above figures give the weights of people who live the longest. (Reprinted courtesy: Metropolitan Life Insurance Co.)

How Many Calories Do You Need?

Next, you need to know the number of calories you require to sustain your present weight. To calculate this, multiply your current weight by ten; this figure is the number of calories your basal metabolism requires to run your basic body processes. Increase this figure by 30 percent to account for your various physical activities. If you exercise regularly, refer to Table 1 (page 21) to find out how many calories you use during your workouts; add that figure to your calculations.

For example, if you weigh 150 pounds, the number of calories you need each day to keep your body running is:

150 × 10 = 1,500 calories

Your caloric requirement for usual physical activities (walking, moving, etc.) is:

1,500 × .3 = 450 calories

The calories required to maintain your weight plus the amount needed for usual physical activities:

1,500 + 450 = 1,950 calories

If you also workout for fifteen minutes on a rowing machine each day, you would add another 105 calories (see Table 1), so your total daily needs would be:

1,950 + 105 = 2,055 calories

The Metabolic "Catch"

Now that you know how many calories you need to maintain your present weight, you have to know how much you have to eliminate to lose the weight you want. As we said, to take off one pound in a week you must either reduce your caloric intake by 3,500 calories or increase your energy expenditure (through exercise) by 3,500 calories. If you're going to lose the pound by dieting alone, you might think that all you have to do is reduce your daily intake by 500 calories. If you use 300 calories in an exercise program, then you can surely reach that goal by eliminating 200 calories' worth of food—a few potatoes perhaps, or a slice of meat, right? Unfortunately, wrong.

This is the metabolic "catch." It works in the beginning, but you'll soon stop losing weight. Why? Because after two or three weeks of dieting the body adjusts to a lower caloric intake by lowering its metabolic rate. Your body actually resists weight changes. It responds to the diet as if you were starving and comes to the rescue by using calories more efficiently in order to maintain your original weight. This is called its "set point." By three weeks into the diet, your body is working at 30 percent greater efficiency, its maximum. This is enough to prevent you from losing any more weight.

How the Paris Diet Eliminates This Problem

The Paris Diet overcomes the set point by changing your caloric levels and tricking your body. For example, if you are a light eater, first you increase what you eat to get your body's efficiency rate back to normal. You see, if you've been dieting all your life or just eating too little, your metabolism is working so efficiently you'd virtually have to starve to lose weight. By first eating a 1,200-calorie, then a 1,400-calorie diet (the Preparation Program), your body will return to a sensible level of efficiency. Since the foods included in this program are high in protein, you won't gain any extra weight even though you're eating more. Some people even lose a few pounds.

The next phase of the diet for light eaters, and the first stage for almost everyone else, is the Weight Loss Program—a diet that starts at only 600 calories. At this level your body will attempt to become more efficient. But just about everyone loses weight at this caloric level since it is only enough to maintain a person weighing about fifty pounds. No matter how much the body tries to slow down its metabolism, it can't compensate enough: Remember, 30 percent is as efficient as it gets.

Even when a diet consists of gourmet food, 600 calories is very little to eat. So you then graduate to the second stage of the Weight Loss Program, the 900-calorie level. Now the body becomes a little less efficient, speeds up its metabolism, and burns off more calories to compensate for the higher level. By the time it has adapted to this level, you graduate to the Adjustment Program, at a 1,200-calorie level, and the body becomes less efficient again. You continue to lose weight.

Once you get down to your ideal weight, you must maintain it for at least a month in order to change your set point permanently to a new level. Once that new point is achieved, the body will defend it by adjusting its rate of efficiency. Even if you slip here and there, you won't gain any extra pounds.

Although this may seem like a slow process, it's the only way to take weight off and to keep it off. Other diets can cause a dramatic loss of weight in the beginning but then do nothing after a few weeks. Or the weight comes off but it's gained back once the diet stops. If you go on and off diets repeatedly, the body becomes more and more resistant to any type of weight loss. It becomes a frustrating ordeal. You may have reached a point where you can't lose anything no matter how little you eat.

But the situation is no longer hopeless. You are holding the solution right in your hands.

———————— ✤ ————————

CHAPTER 3

How to Follow
the Paris Diet

*B*y now you're probably anxious to get started. This chapter will give you what you need first—a personal dieting schedule.

The Paris Diet is designed for all types of people with different metabolisms, caloric requirements, and weight loss needs. Certain groups must follow it in certain ways. The following is an easy reference summary to the entire diet. First, you'll have to determine which type of eater you are. Second, you must decide how much you want to lose. Then follow the program that fits your needs, exactly as it's described here. You can't fail!

You will notice that some of the plans have long and short versions. Although the diet works well in its short form, we have found that the long version is most likely to keep the unwanted weight off permanently.* It's up to you. If you want to take weight off more quickly, follow the short program; if you want extra assurance that you'll never gain it back, take the long route. The more time you give your body to adjust to each caloric level, the more your new weight will be set.

Whichever plan you follow or whatever time frame you choose, you'll be pleased with the results. Just don't shorten or lengthen any stage of the diet beyond what we've indicated.

To demonstrate how the diet works and how much weight you can expect to lose, we have included case studies. Because of individ-

---

* The reason why the last two programs don't have a long and short version is because they apply to very heavy eaters whose weight will be reduced effectively by this type of caloric restriction, without the need to extend the plan.

ual differences in size, energy expenditure, and metabolic rate, your own weight loss may be different. A person who sits at a desk all day will not lose as much as someone who exercises every afternoon. For this reason, our examples come from average cases. (Our cases are drawn from the short versions of the plans to give you an idea of what you can expect without taking up too much space.)

The Life-Dieter Plan

If you:

are a light eater (under 1,400 calories daily), or
are always dieting, or
dieted less than two months ago, you should follow this diet schedule:

SHORT PLAN	PHASE OF DIET	LONG PLAN
2 wk	Preparation Program: Stage One	3–4 wk
2 wk	Preparation Program: Stage Two	3–4 wk
2 wk	Weight Loss Program: Stage One	3 wk
2 wk	Weight Loss Program: Stage Two	2 wk
2 wk	Adjustment Program: Stage One	2 wk
2 wk	Adjustment Program: Stage Two	1 mo
2 wk	Maintenance Program: Stage One	1 mo
2 wk +	Maintenance Program: Stage Two	1 mo +

EXAMPLE: Catherine P. is a forty-seven-year-old woman who is five feet five inches tall, and when she came to us, weighed 155 pounds. Because she is near menopause, it is easier for her to gain weight and harder for her to lose it. Catherine has had a weight problem for quite some time and so has carefully watched her food intake. In fact, she has been on some type of restricted diet since her thirties (when she first gained an extra fifteen pounds), rarely eating more than 1,000 calories a day. Recently, in spite of her life-dieting habit, she gained another ten pounds. That was when she decided to try the Paris Diet. While on the life-dieter plan, she showed the following losses:

WEEK	AMOUNT OF WEIGHT LOST (lb)
1	2
2	1
3	0
4	0
5	8
6	5
7	4
8	3
9	2
10	1
11	1
12	1
13	0
14	0
15	no weight gain
16 +	no weight gain

In all, Catherine lost twenty-eight pounds and was able to eat 1,800 calories a day on the Maintenance Program without gaining any weight back.

The Over-Twenty Pound Weight Loss Plan

If you are:

a large person, or
an average to healthy eater (1,500–2,500 calories daily), and
more than twenty pounds overweight:

SHORT PLAN	PHASE OF DIET	LONG PLAN
2 wk	Weight Loss Program: Stage One	3 wk
2 wk	Weight Loss Program: Stage Two	2 wk
2 wk	Adjustment Program: Stage One	2 wk
2 wk	Adjustment Program: Stage Two	1 mo
2 wk	Maintenance Program: Stage One	1 mo
2 wk	Maintenance Program: Stage Two	1 mo +
2–4 wk	Maintenance Program: Stage Three*	1 mo

* For heavy eaters and those who consume 1,400–2,000 calories.

If you are more than thirty pounds overweight, you may have to
follow this program twice. If so, you must first stay on 2,000 calories
(the Maintenance Program) for at least one month before starting
over again.

EXAMPLE: Lili L, thirty-two, had been overweight since adolescence.
She carefully followed a restricted diet five years ago and lost weight
but gained everything back while on the "maintenance program" of
that plan. When she came to us, she was five feet five inches tall and
weighed 190 pounds. Lili never was a life-dieter. She enjoyed her
food and often ate 2,000–2,400 calories per day. Therefore, we put
her on this plan, where she lost:

WEEK	AMOUNT OF WEIGHT LOST (lb)
1	10
2	5
3	5
4	5
5	4
6	3
7	1
8	1
9	1
10	1
11	0
12	0

On this first cycle, Lili lost thirty-six pounds. She stayed at the 2,000-calorie level for two months, then started the program again. The second time around she lost an additional twenty-five pounds (on the second cycle people tend to lose about two-thirds of what they lost on the first). Lili is now down to the weight she wants.

The Twenty Pound or Under Weight Loss Plan

If you are:

a large person, or
an average to healthy eater (1,500–2,500 calories daily), and
twenty pounds or less overweight:

SHORT PLAN	PHASE OF DIET	LONG PLAN
2 wk	Adjustment Program: Stage One	2 wk
2 wk	Adjustment Program: Stage Two	1 mo
2 wk	Maintenance Program: Stage One	1 mo
2 wk +	Maintenance Program: Stage Two	1 mo
2–4 wk	Maintenance Program: Stage Three*	1 mo +

* For heavy eaters and those who consume 1,400–2,000 calories.

EXAMPLE: Gerard B., a forty-five-year-old businessman who is not very active, had gained twenty pounds in six months. (Because of a promotion, he was attending lavish business lunches.) Six feet tall, he weighed 190 pounds when he came to us. He wanted to weigh 170 again. We found that he was an average eater and drinker, consuming about 2,400 calories per day. This was how the program worked for him:

WEEK	AMOUNT OF WEIGHT LOST (lb)
1	5
2	3
3	3
4	3
5	2
6	2
7	1
8	0

Gerard lost nineteen pounds without any trouble and loved the gourmet food he prepared from the Chef's Recipes. He now eats a healthier version of the amount he did before and doesn't gain weight.

The Hearty Eater Plan

If you are:

a hearty eater (2,500–3,000 calories daily), and
twenty pounds overweight:

	PHASE OF DIET
2 wk	Adjustment Program: Stage One
2 wk	Adjustment Program: Stage Two
2 wk	Maintenance Program: Stage One
2 wk	Maintenance Program: Stage Two
2 wk	Maintenance Program: Stage Three

If you need to lose more weight after this ten-week program, wait at least one month at 2,000 calories, then start again but with the Weight Loss Program. The second cycle of this plan would be:

2 wk	Weight Loss Program: Stage One
2 wk	Weight Loss Program: Stage Two
2 wk	Adjustment Program: Stage One
2 wk	Adjustment Program: Stage Two
2 wk	Maintenance Program: Stage One
2 wk	Maintenance Program: Stage Two
2–4 wk	Maintenance Program: Stage Three

EXAMPLE: Gerard's boss, Henri D., came to see us after noting his employee's success. He had much the same profile as Gerard, except that he was a larger man and a heavier eater (about 3,000 calories per day). His weight loss chart looked like this:

WEEK	AMOUNT OF WEIGHT LOST (lb)
1	6
2	4
3	4
4	3
5	3
6	2
7	1
8	1
9	1
10	0

Henri lost twenty-five pounds and loved the diet. Since he had more to lose, he went through the program again, starting with the Weight Loss Program. By the end of the second cycle, he had lost another twenty pounds, achieving his ideal weight for a man six feet two inches tall.

The Heavy Eater Plan

If you are:

a very heavy eater (more than 3,000 calories daily), and
twenty pounds overweight:

	PHASE OF DIET
2 wk	Adjustment Program: Stage Two
2 wk	Maintenance Program: Stage One
2 wk	Maintenance Program: Stage Two
2 wk	Maintenance Program: Stage Three

If you need to lose more weight, stay at Stage Three for one month, then start the second cycle with the following schedule:

	PHASE OF DIET
2 wk	Weight Loss Program: Stage One
2 wk	Weight Loss Program: Stage Two
2 wk	Adjustment Program: Stage One
2 wk	Adjustment Program: Stage Two
2 wk	Maintenance Program: Stage One
2 wk	Maintenance Program: Stage Two
2 wk	Maintenance Program: Stage Three

EXAMPLE: Paul H., thirty-seven, is a prominent French attorney who came to us because he had gained twenty pounds in three years. He is five feet ten inches and weighed 180 pounds. Before this, he had exercised frequently, but his recent workload had not left him with many free hours for tennis or workouts. He was a big eater, often consuming over 3,000 calories per day. We told him the good news: Since he ate so much, he didn't have to follow any of the low-calorie stages. His personal record is as follows:

	AMOUNT OF
WEEK	WEIGHT LOST (lb)
1	6
2	4
3	4
4	3
5	3
6	2
7	1
8	1

Paul lost twenty-four pounds and recommended the diet to all his clients!

You may be wondering how many calories you really eat each day. One way to find out is to keep an exact record of one week's meals (a sample food diary for you to copy and use follows on page 40). Show this to a dietician, doctor, or nutritionist. He or she will then calculate your daily caloric intake. If you can't or don't want to do this, that's fine too. You can estimate. Light eaters start with the Life-Dieter Plan, normal eaters with either the Over Twenty Pound Weight Loss Plan or the Twenty Pound or Under Weight Loss Plan, and big eaters with The Hearty Eater Plan.

―――――― ✦ ――――――

CHAPTER 4

How to Make
the Paris Diet
Work for You

*Y*ou're now ready to embark on an exciting food adventure that will change your life—the Paris Diet. It will open up a whole new world of delicious ways to choose and prepare food. It will take off your excess weight easily and quickly and train your body never to gain weight again. Because of the foods you'll be eating, you will feel healthier and have more energy, your skin and hair will look better than ever before, and your body will be in excellent shape.

Before you begin, there are some essential tips you must know in order to get the most out of the program. These guidelines will tell you how to eat in every situation, how to prepare your food, and how to season it the French way so that even the simplest meals are indescribably delicious.

These tips can be used for all stages of the program. Refer to them each time you start a new stage.

Before You Start, Keep a Food Diary

Before you start the diet, you need to know how much you eat. Then you can decide which of the dieting plans described in this chapter is the right one for you. Eat as you normally do for a week before beginning the diet, and write down *everything* you take in, including even the smallest of snacks. After you've completed this record, take it to your doctor, dietitian, or nutritionist to learn how many calories you consume each day. (If you want to skip this step and estimate your caloric intake, see the guidelines in Chapter 3.)

You can photocopy the following sample page and use it for your personal food diary:

Sample Food Diary

NAME: _____

DATE: _____ DAY OF THE WEEK: _____

BREAKFAST (INCLUDE AMOUNTS OF ALL FOODS AND BEVERAGES
FOR EVERY MEAL): _____

_____

_____

_____

MIDMORNING SNACK: _____

_____

LUNCH: _____

_____

_____

AFTERNOON SNACK: _____

_____

DINNER: _____

_____

_____

_____

EVENING SNACK: _____

_____

ANY OTHER FOOD OR DRINK: _____

_____

_____

_____

_____

Know How and When to Weigh Yourself

Weighing yourself every day can be discouraging except at the beginning of the Weight Loss Program. During that phase, seeing how quickly you shed extra pounds should motivate you to stick with it. The body normally goes through slight daily fluctuations in weight. Weighing in each morning during the other phases of the diet may be misleading. Women, for instance, can put on between one and five pounds before their periods and lose it immediately afterward.

When you weigh yourself, do it before breakfast, after going to the toilet. Make sure you wear the same clothes (or no clothes), and use the same scale. Record the date and your weight on a copy of the Weight Record Chart, which follows.

Here is a schedule of how you should record your weight during the four phases of the diet. If you start with the Weight Loss Program, begin by weighing yourself every day; if you start with the Adjustment Program, weigh yourself once a week.

Weigh Yourself Before You Start.

Preparation Program:	Once a week (usually on Monday)
Weight Loss Program, First Week:	Every day
Weight Loss Program, Second Week:	Twice a week (usually on Mondays and Thursdays)
Weight Loss Program, Third Week:	Twice a week
Weight Loss Program, Fourth Week:	Once a week
Adjustment and Maintenance Programs:	Once a week

Photocopy the following sample page to record your weight:

Weight Record Chart

Shorter Plan

THE PREPARATION PROGRAM

First Week	_____ lb
Second Week	_____ lb
Third Week	_____ lb
Fourth Week	_____ lb

THE WEIGHT LOSS PROGRAM

First Week	Monday	_____ lb
	Tuesday	_____ lb
	Wednesday	_____ lb
	Thursday	_____ lb
	Friday	_____ lb
	Saturday	_____ lb
	Sunday	_____ lb
Second Week	Monday	_____ lb
	Thursday	_____ lb
Third Week	Monday	_____ lb
	Thursday	_____ lb
Fourth Week		_____ lb

THE ADJUSTMENT PROGRAM

First Week	_____ lb
Second Week	_____ lb
Third Week	_____ lb
Fourth Week	_____ lb

THE MAINTENANCE PROGRAM

First Week	_____ lb
Second Week	_____ lb
Third Week	_____ lb
Fourth Week	_____ lb

WEIGHT AT START OF PROGRAM   _____ lb
WEIGHT AT END OF PROGRAM   _____ lb

Weight Record Chart

Long Plan

THE PREPARATION PROGRAM

First Week	_____ lb	Fifth Week	_____ lb
Second Week	_____ lb	Sixth Week	_____ lb
Third Week	_____ lb	Seventh Week	_____ lb
Fourth Week	_____ lb	Eighth Week	_____ lb

THE WEIGHT LOSS PROGRAM

First Week	M _____ lb	Fourth Week	M _____ lb
	T _____ lb		Th _____ lb
	W _____ lb	Fifth Week	M _____ lb
	Th _____ lb		Th _____ lb
	F _____ lb	Sixth Week	_____ lb
	Sa _____ lb	Seventh Week	_____ lb
	S _____ lb	Eighth Week	_____ lb
Second Week	M _____ lb		
	Th _____ lb		
Third Week	M _____ lb		
	Th _____ lb		

THE ADJUSTMENT PROGRAM

First Week	_____ lb	Fifth Week	_____ lb
Second Week	_____ lb	Sixth Week	_____ lb
Third Week	_____ lb	Seventh Week	_____ lb
Fourth Week	_____ lb	Eighth Week	_____ lb

THE MAINTENANCE PROGRAM

First Week	_____ lb	Fifth Week	_____ lb
Second Week	_____ lb	Sixth Week	_____ lb
Third Week	_____ lb	Seventh Week	_____ lb
Fourth Week	_____ lb	Eighth Week	_____ lb

WEIGHT AT START OF PROGRAM _____ lb
WEIGHT AT END OF PROGRAM _____ lb

Develop Good Eating Habits

Many people sabotage their efforts to lose weight with bad eating habits. If this applies to you, it's time to develop new and healthy habits. Once you begin the diet and forever afterward:

eat three meals a day, preferably at a set time,

never skip a meal (if you do, your protein needs will not be taken care of, your hunger will increase, and nibbling could result),

don't wait until you're starving to eat (when you're very hungry, you usually eat more than you should),

eat sitting down and take your time,

chew your food slowly and carefully,

try to eat in a well-lit, comfortable room that pleases your senses,

don't nibble between meals and while preparing them,

don't compare yourself to very thin or much younger people—find your ideal weight (Table 2, page 26), and make that your goal,

don't snack; meditate, exercise, or try some other relaxation techniques to overcome nervous eating,

don't "taste" leftovers or sample foods at the specialty store,

don't exceed the amount of foods listed in the Paris Diet, or substitute foods that are not on the menus or exchange tables—you might think that one food is just like another or that "a little extra can't hurt," but it can contain a lot more calories than you think.

Don't Systematically Weigh Your Food

It's important to weigh your food when you begin the diet so that you can stick to the amounts indicated. You'll soon know what 4 ounces of fish look like. Weighing food each time you eat can be tedious. Besides, although we say that a diet contains x number of calories, there is always a slight variation over or under that amount. If your piece of fish really weighs 6¹/₁₀ ounces, it isn't going to make that much of a difference.

Don't Add Extra Salt to Your Meals

Especially during the Weight Loss Program, don't add any extra salt to your meals. Some of our recipes have salt just to keep your taste buds satisfied, but don't add any more. Some people who eat too much salt during a weekend—believe it or not—gain six to eight pounds! There's nothing more depressing than discovering during a Monday morning weigh-in that you've regained what you lost after a week's worth of dieting almost overnight. Although it's water weight and not fat and will eventually be eliminated, your sense of achievement and gratification are threatened.

Many processed foods have "hidden" ingredients, so read labels carefully to see if salt (or sodium) is mentioned among the first few items. Fast foods can be notoriously high in salt. For a complete list of sodium-rich foods, see Table 3. You will notice that some of these foods are included in the diet: We've allowed for these. But you must not add more than what's indicated.

TABLE 3
Sodium-Rich Foods

FOOD	SERVING SIZE	SODIUM (mg)
bacon, broiled	3 oz	875
beans, baked	1 cup	860
beans, lima	1 cup	190
beets, canned	1 cup	380
bread, rye	1 slice	139
bread, white	1 slice	128
bread, whole wheat	1 slice	150
butter, salted	1 oz	280
catsup	1 tbs	160
cheese, American	1 oz	405
cheese, bleu	1 oz	450
cheese, Camembert	1 oz	290
cheese, Cheddar	1 oz	176
cheese, feta	1 oz	316
cheese, Monterey Jack	1 oz	150
cheese, mozzarella, whole milk	1 oz	150

FOOD	SERVING SIZE	SODIUM (mg)
cheese, Parmesan	1 oz	210
cheese, Provolone	1 oz	250
chicken, cooked	4 oz	75–100
clams, cooked	4 oz	140
corn, canned	1 cup	500
cornflakes	1 oz	300
crab, cooked	4 oz	1,150
fish, cooked	4 oz	125–200
garlic salt	1 tsp	1,900
ham, cooked	4 oz	1,063
horseradish, grated	1 tbs	200
lobster, cooked	4 oz	240
margarine	1 oz	280
meat tenderizer	1 tsp	1,750
MSG (monosodium glutamate)	1 tsp	490
olives, green	4 medium	390
onion salt	1 tsp	1,600
peanut butter	1 oz	170
peas, canned	1 cup	400
pickles, dill	1	850
pretzels	1	270
relish	1 tbs	125
salad dressing	1 tbs	100–330
sardines, cooked	4 oz	940
sauce, barbeque	1 tbs	130
sauce, chili	1 tbs	230
sauce, soy	1 tbs	1,030
sauce, tartar	1 tbs	180
sauce, Worcestershire	1 tbs	200
sausage, cooked	4 oz	1,095
tomato juice	1 cup	485
turkey, roast	4 oz	150

Drink Plenty of Fluids

If you've dieted before, you've heard this already. On high protein plans it's especially important to flush out the body. Make sure you drink at least six to ten glasses of water each day. Add lemon juice or herbs for flavor, or substitute mineral water (carbonated or not), coffee, or tea. Drink low-calorie soft drinks only occasionally, as a treat, but never between meals: Low-calorie drinks make you feel hungry and increase your cravings for sugar.

Until You Reach the Maintenance Stage, Don't Drink Alcohol

During the Preparation, Weight Loss, and Adjustment Programs, you must not drink any alcohol. Alcoholic beverages contain very high calorie levels (see Table 4). You'll be able to drink—although in moderation—once you reach the Maintenance Program.

Until You Reach the Maintenance Stage, Avoid Sugar and Sweet Flavorings

Do not add sugar or syrupy flavorings to yogurt, cottage cheese, fruits, coffee, tea, etc. Artificial sweeteners are permitted.

Remember: Men Differ from Women in Many Ways

Vive la différence! And when following the same diet, men usually lose more weight than women. Because their bodies use up more energy, men can also eat larger portions, drink more alcohol, and enjoy richer foods without putting on the same number of pounds.

If a man only has a few pounds to lose, he doesn't have to follow the Weight Loss Program. The protein-rich 1,200 or 1,400 calorie diets will allow him to shed seven to eleven pounds within a few weeks.

TABLE 4
Caloric Content of Alcoholic Drinks

DRINK	SERVING SIZE	CALORIES
anisette	⅔ oz	74
beer	8 oz	100
beer, ale	8 oz	98
beer, light	8 oz	70

DRINK	SERVING SIZE	CALORIES
Benedictine	⅔ oz	70
Bloody Mary	3½ oz	105
brandy, apricot	1 oz	96
brandy Alexander	3½ oz	280
brandy, California	1 oz	73
champagne	4 oz	85
cider	4 oz	50
cognac	1 oz	73
crème de menthe	⅔ oz	67
curaçao	⅔ oz	54
daiquiri	3½ oz	120
eggnog	4 oz	335
gin	1½ oz	98–105
grasshopper, with cream	3½ oz	310
Mai-Tai	3½ oz	210
Manhattan	3½ oz	165
margarita	3½ oz	210
martini	3½ oz	140
mint julep	10 oz	210
muscatel, port	4 oz	180
piña colada	3½ oz	200
planter's punch	4 oz	175
rum	1½ oz	115
screwdriver	3½ oz	140
sherry, cooking	4 oz	40
sherry, domestic	4 oz	170
Tom Collins	3½ oz	230
vermouth, French	3½ oz	105
vermouth, Italian	3½ oz	170
vodka	1½ oz	125
whiskey	1½ oz	100–112
whiskey sour	3½ oz	230
wine cooler	12 oz	220
wines, dessert	4 oz	140–160
wines, light	5 oz	65
wines, table	4 oz	100–120

Use the Exchange Tables

In each stage of the diet, you will find exchange tables, also called equivalency tables, which are lists of foods that equal approximately the same calories. To vary your diet—and this is advisable since boredom sabotages any regimen—select a food from these lists that equals the one in the plan. When you substitute another food, don't change the quantity recommended. For example, if you don't feel like having ½ cup of beets, exchange it for 6 ounces of tomato juice; not 4 or 8 ounces, but 6 ounces.

You can also make two exchanges; for instance, if you want to eat an apple, you can exchange it for 10 cherries plus ½ cup of orange juice. Be imaginative!

Not all foods in the menu plans will have exchanges.

Use Supplements During the Weight Loss Program

During the Weight Loss Program, we want to make sure your body is getting all the nutrients it needs. Therefore, take a regular one-per-day multivitamin and mineral supplement containing approximately the amounts of nutrients advised in the Recommended Dietary Allowances (RDA) tables (see page 318) plus a daily supplement of 500 mg of potassium. Women, in particular, should also take a daily supplement of 1,000 mg of calcium to keep their bones strong. During the other stages of the diet, women may continue taking calcium if they choose, and both men and women may continue with the daily multivitamin and nutrient supplement. During these phases of the diet, no extra potassium is needed.

Don't Begin Dieting Immediately Before or During a Vacation or Holiday

Some people believe that kicking any habit—from cigarettes to food —is easier when you're away. Experience has shown us that this just isn't true, especially when it comes to diets. People don't want to follow a weight loss regimen when they're trying to relax. What, after all, is a vacation without a little self-indulgence, without the chance to discover a small country inn with superb cooking or the most fashionable restaurant in town? If you want to get rid of that extra weight before squeezing into your bikini, do it before you go away. Once your weight stabilizes (during the Adjustment and Maintenance Programs), you can go on vacation and occasionally splurge —it's all part of the fun.

It's also a bad idea to start the Weight Loss Program just before holidays such as Christmas or Thanksgiving. If you've really made up your mind to lose weight, it'll hold for another day or two.

Avoid Snacking; But If You Can't, Use Only Our Suggestions

As a rule, we do not encourage any type of snacking on the Paris Diet for several reasons. First of all, the foods are carefully calculated, and any additional calories could sabotage all your efforts. For example, let's say you're on the Weight Loss Program and are tempted to eat a few peanuts in the afternoon. Those nuts could add an extra 100 calories to your daily intake and throw the whole plan off.

But the second problem with snacking is far simpler: It's a bad habit you should kick once and for all. Too many weight problems stem not so much from what is eaten at meals, but from what is eaten between meals. Some of our patients, without even realizing it, have added as much as 500 to 1,000 calories per day from snacking.

If you need an extra "something," and exercising or meditating won't do the trick, here are some suggestions:

1. Save a dessert from lunch or dinner and have it for a snack. Just remember not to have it twice. For example, if you eat a piece of fruit between meals, remove it from the dinner menu of that day.

2. Cold water with lemon or carbonated water is a good hunger-quencher.

3. Choose a snack from this list of "free" foods. These are items with almost no caloric value. They can be used in unlimited quantitites on everything but the first stage of the Weight Loss Program. For that phase, stick to the above suggestions.

"Free" Foods for Snacking
(except for Weight Loss Program: Stage One)

bouillon (without salt)
chicory
Chinese cabbage
clear broth
coffee
endive
escarole
gelatin (unsweetened)

lemon
lettuce (all kinds)
lime
parsley
popcorn (plain, no
    salt, butter, or
    cheese)

radishes
tea
vinegar
water
watercress

Advice for Choosing and Preparing Food

Caloric value can be influenced as much by the way you prepare food as the amount you eat. Cooking with oils or fats can almost double the number of calories in a meal.

Remember: to eat right, you don't have to sacrifice taste. No nation prides itself on its cuisine more than the French. Even during the strict phases of the program, your food can still be delicious and satisfying. Unless otherwise indicated by our recipes, stick to the following cooking and preparation methods.

ALL FOODS should be lightly salted and cooked with little or no fat.

AVOID heavily salted, sweetened, creamed, or processed foods. Check labels for ingredients. Use fresh foods whenever possible; if you must use canned or frozen ingredients, check the label to make sure no sugar or salt is added. Avoid prepared frozen "diet" meals since they normally contain too little protein in relation to their caloric content and surprisingly contain starches and fats that you shouldn't have on lower calorie diets.

MEATS should be:

> skinless (poultry) and trimmed of fat
> grilled on a grill or in a nonstick pan
> cooked in a regular or microwave oven
> cooked in a rotisserie (chicken, roasts)

boiled (lean beef, stewing veal)
cooked in sealed aluminum foil (rabbit, skinned and boned
    turkey, chicken breasts)

VEGETABLES should be:

fresh
canned, packed in water only
frozen, uncooked, no salt added
boiled
steamed
cooked in a regular or microwave oven

FRUITS should be:

fresh
if canned, packed in its own juice, no sugar added
if frozen, unsweetened, for making purées
baked, chopped, or diced

SOUPS should be:

thin, such as consommé
unsalted
not chunky or creamed

COTTAGE CHEESE or YOGURT may be eaten:

low fat, plain, without sugar, artificially sweetened
with chopped or puréed fruit, but according to your daily
    allowance only
with pepper, herbs, or spices

Advice for Using Spices, Herbs, and Condiments the French Way

Much of what makes French food so delicious is the way it's sea-
soned. You normally may use seasonings in a different way, and that's
fine, too. Here are some secrets for preparing and using these ingredients from some of the finest French chefs.

BASIL: raw only, do not cook

For pasta or cottage cheese: purée and blend in.

Use on the Following Foods: pasta, salads, ratatouille, zucchini, baked tomatoes, green peas, chicken, sautéed veal, red snapper, cottage cheese.

BAY LEAVES: use only 2 or 3 leaves; powder to sprinkle

Use on the Following Foods: tomatoes, ratatouille, cabbage, roast pork, mussels, in tomato sauce.

CLOVES: whole, inserted into food

Use on the Following Foods: baked apple or apple purée, lentils, carrots, baked ham.

CORIANDER: grind the seed for all uses except in soups, where you should use the leaves only

Use on the Following Foods: consommés, lentils, ratatouille, tomatoes, beans, rice, raw mushrooms, roasted meats, marmalade.

DILL: chopped with scissors

Use on the Following Foods: soups, salads, all vegetables, scrambled eggs, white fish such as sole, in vinaigrettes or tomato sauces.

FENNEL: do not overcook or it loses its flavor

Use on the Following Foods: scallops, pork, chicken.

GARLIC: raw or cooked

For meat: slit the thickest part with a knife and insert into the meat ½ clove cut vertically before roasting.

For vegetables: finely chopped.

For cottage cheese: puréed and blended into cottage cheese.

Note: To remove any odor from your breath, crunch a grain of coffee in your mouth after eating garlic.

Use on the Following Foods: ratatouille, mushrooms, tomatoes, roast lamb or pork, veal, spaghetti, cottage cheese.

GINGER: powdered or grated, sprinkled

Use on the Following Foods: melon, fruit salad, rice, chicken, fish soup.

LEMON: use thin slices as garnish; thicker slices or a few drops of juice for flavor

Use on the Following Foods: fish, salads, in beverages.

MINT: use leaves for decoration; powder for taste
Use on the Following Foods: cucumber, lamb, chicken, cottage cheese, in vinaigrette and fruit salads.

MUSTARD: regular, in moderation (prepared mustards are high in salt)
Use on the Following Foods: with mayonnaise, in vinaigrette, on all cold meats.

NUTMEG: grated
Use on the Following Foods: pasta, beans, potatoes, spinach, cauliflower, poached or scrambled eggs, pork, veal, cottage cheese.

ONIONS: cooked only
Use on the Following Foods: vegetables, rice.

PARSLEY: chopped
  On salad greens: raw
  On all other foods: cooked
Use on the Following Foods: soups, salads, meat, all vegetables, pasta, in vinaigrette.

PEPPER: ground, sprinkle powder
Use on the Following Foods: soup, salads, all vegetables, pasta, beans, potatoes, sauces, grilled fish or meat, cottage cheese, eggs.

SAFFRON: powdered, sprinkle sparingly
Use on the Following Foods: rice, fish soup.

SHALLOTS: raw or cooked, chopped
Use on the Following Foods: salads, fish, in vinaigrette (with lemon), cottage cheese.

TABASCO SAUCE: a few drops
Use on the Following Foods: soup, salads, tomato juice (with lemon), in sauces.

TARRAGON: dry powder, sprinkled over food
Use on the Following Foods: soups, salads, peas, tomatoes, grilled chicken, roast veal or pork, in vinaigrette.

VANILLA: for dairy products
  bean: during boiling
  powder: sprinkle
  extract: a few drops
Use on the Following Foods: rice pudding, cream of wheat, crèmes.

Add Salad Dressings and Sauces Whenever You Can

We have included recipes (see the section starting on page 241) for fourteen dressings and sauces that can be used to add to the flavor and texture of salads, vegetables, and main dishes. Do not add your own or any store-bought dressings that contain over 25 calories per tablespoon.

During Stage One of the Weight Loss Program, you can make a light dressing/sauce with lemon juice, herbs, pepper, vinegar, and a small chopped onion (approximately 5 calories per tablespoon). Sauces can be made from puréed vegetables. Reduce tomatoes, eggplants, mushrooms, watercress, celery, leeks, and/or diced carrots to a pulp through long, slow cooking; flavor with spices and herbs, and then use to season dishes (about 5 calories per tablespoon). You can also use the following recipes (page numbers are in parentheses):

FOR SALADS
Sauce Verte/Green Dressing (page 252)
Sauce Menthe/Mint Vinegar (page 248)
Sauce Sontay/Creamy Spinach Dressing (page 249)
Sauce Yogourt/Yogurt Sauce (page 249)
Sauce Tomates aux Aromates/Spicy Tomato Sauce (page 253)
Vinaigre Zéro/Red Vinaigrette (page 247)

FOR VEGETABLES AND FISH
Sauce Maraîchère/Tomato and Lemon Sauce with Herbs (page 253)

FOR ZUCCHINI, COLD MEAT, AND FISH
Sauce Tomates à la Chinoise/Chinese-Style Tomato Sauce (page 254)

During Stage Two of the Weight Loss Program, you can use all of the dressings and sauces listed above, plus these extras:

FOR SALADS
Sauce Roquefort/Roquefort Cheese Dressing (page 252)
Sauce Grande Bêche/Watercress Dressing (page 250)

FOR SALADS, POULTRY, VEAL, AND BOILED FISH
Sauce Aïoli/Creamed Garlic Dressing (page 250)

During the Preparation and Adjustment Programs (both stages), you can use all of the sauces/dressings listed above, plus:

FOR SALADS, POULTRY, AND VEAL
Sauce Provençale/Vinaigrette with Tarragon (page 248)

FOR EGGPLANT, ZUCCHINI, AND PASTA
Sauce Saint-Jeannet/Piperade Dressing (page 251)
On the 1,200 calorie plan, you can also use regular salad dressings once a day; on 1,400 calories and up you can use regular salad dressings twice a day.
During each phase of the diet, we will repeat the dressings and sauces you can use for that plan.

Life Goes on Even When You Diet

There's a French saying that roughly translates: If you don't like something, you don't have to put others off it. Just because *you* can't have pastrami, pecan pie, or a drink, doesn't mean they've stopped tasting good to the people around you. The best way to get your family, friends, and coworkers to help you is to avoid criticizing their bad eating habits. They were probably yours only a few weeks ago!

If you overpromote a diet, some people may want to sabotage it. It's sad to say, but this is human nature. They'll tell you how your meals aren't well-balanced (untrue), or how you looked better before (you know this isn't true), or that friends on different diets lost more weight more quickly. (They probably gained back the weight just as quickly as they lost it.) Your diet is your business, so tell only those people you know will be supportive.

You may want to tell co-workers so that they won't tempt you with butter cookies or chocolates. If possible, it's certainly worth getting support from friends and family, who can provide encouragement if you weaken.

If you want to motivate your loved ones gently toward healthier eating habits, pin the Chef's Menu up in the kitchen. Pretty soon they'll be begging for those better-balanced meals!

If You're Single

It's often a chore to cook for yourself. We know how some singles cook: a hamburger eaten while standing in the kitchen, a couple of cookies, and a bowl of ice cream in front of the television. Sound familiar?

Rediscover the pleasure of eating with the Paris Diet. Sit down to a well-laid table. Get all the ingredients you need a day in advance so that you won't be tempted to heat up a store-bought frozen dinner. Lunch or dinner should be a genuine meal even on the low-calorie plans. It takes less time to prepare a light, satisfying meal than it takes to go back and forth from the living room to the refrigerator.

If you don't like spending time in the kitchen, make double portions of those listed in the recipes. Why not prepare four or eight helpings at a time during the weekend? You can pop them in the freezer in separate serving-size containers or plastic bags. That way, when you come home from work, your gourmet meal can be ready in minutes.

If You Have a Family

It's lovely to think of others, but right now you must think of yourself. You'll have to establish new eating habits with those you love. This doesn't mean that you have to put your whole family on a diet, but it shouldn't be torture for you when the children come home from school and your husband or your wife returns from work. Ask for a few simple favors during the weeks you're on the strict Weight Loss Program. If they're old enough, let the children prepare their own snacks. Ask your husband to avoid having his cocktail or snacking in front of you. If he feels you're determined to stick with this diet, he won't ask you to serve him peanuts or chips.

If your husband does want to diet, he probably won't need to follow the Weight Loss Program (see the guidelines in Chapter 3). As we've already said, children shouldn't follow the diet at all. They're still growing and need hearty meals. Overweight adolescents may be put on a diet of this type, but only under a doctor's strict supervision, and then rarely at the lower caloric stages.

To make your life easier, don't prepare two separate menus; for instance, if you start with raw vegetables, your family can use whatever sauce they like while you squeeze on lemon juice with herbs. There's also nothing to stop you from making the main dish for the whole family from the Paris Diet (they will especially enjoy the recipes from the Chef's Menu), but let them also have their French fries or special rice.

You must avoid nibbling, no easy feat when you're preparing the family meal. Fight the temptation to taste what you're cooking. And don't finish food your child has left on the plate.

Butter or heavy sauces on green beans and other vegetables are out for you, but your family can still enjoy them.

Don't worry about dessert. Your family is bound to love many of the Paris Diet recipes, like Cinnamon-Flavored Strawberries, Low-Calorie Dark Chocolate Mousse, Fruit Skewers, or Baked Apple Surprise. They'll probably ask for them again. If they insist on nibbling in front of the television, save your dessert from dinner to enjoy at the same time.

The French art of eating includes the joy of sharing good food, so your diet should take others into consideration. If your husband or wife does want to lose a few pounds, that's the best situation. You can help each other to stick with it.

If You Visit with Friends

Even when you're dieting, a dinner party can be fun. Why refuse an invitation? A diet doesn't have to be a prison. You don't have to call your hostess and warn her not to include this or that food. You can always find on-the-spot solutions, like raw vegetables, fruit, or salads (with a lemon juice and herb dressing).

Wine and alcohol can be refused graciously. The dangers of smoking and drinking are now apparent, and good friends will not force you to drink. Similarly, you can refuse to nibble and still socialize. When drinks or wine are served, just take some mineral water with a twist of lemon, and stay away from the hors d'oeuvres and peanuts (just fifteen of those small munchies contain 100 calories). For the main course, eat one reasonable helping that fits into your diet. If you still find it hard to socialize and follow the program, confide in your host or hostess when you arrive. Many people today are on diets and work out to keep in shape. They'll understand, and may even help you not to slip.

If You Have to Go to a Restaurant

This really should be a breeze since you're the one who selects the food. If you're on the strict Weight Loss Program, order a salad with a lemon juice and herb dressing for starters and some grilled shrimp with a vegetable (no butter) as the main dish. Either ask for food without sauces or request them dry and grilled, with dressings or sauces on the side (then don't use them). Avoid creamy or chunky soups. If you haven't eaten any fruit for breakfast or lunch, select a mixed fruit salad for dessert.

Always order grilled or poached fish rather than meat if you have the choice. Fish is leaner than the leanest of meats, and restaurants tend to use the fattier cuts of meats (like filet mignon) because they have more flavor.

When you graduate to the higher calorie stages of the plan, you'll have a much larger choice and can eat like anyone else at the table, as well as drink one or two glasses of wine.

If You Are Entertaining at Home

Having guests is even easier than eating out since you're the one in charge. For a light first course, prepare a salad (with one of our special dressings) or small grilled shrimp. A main dish can be selected from the Chef's Recipes. End the meal with cheese and a Chef's dessert.

If your friends comment on how delicious the meal was, tell them it was from a diet. The next time you visit their house for dinner, you may find that they're on the Paris Diet, too.

Use The Right Exercise for
Each Stage of the Diet

We have designed a special exercise program (Chapter 12) that perfectly complements the Paris Diet. If you want to use your own
exercises, follow our guidelines in that chapter. For example, during
the Weight Loss Program, you shouldn't do any sort of strenuous
exercise. You are not eating enough calories to provide you with the
energy you need. During this stage, do only simple stretching and
toning exercises. For the Preparation and Adjustment Programs, use
regular types of exercise, but again, nothing too strenuous. Only
during the Maintenance Program, (1,600 calories and above) should
you start doing heavy workouts.

By all means, exercise at least three times a week for at least fifteen
to twenty minutes. Exercise tones up and strengthens the body,
improves your health, aids in weight loss, and gives you a boost of
energy.

How to Use the Paris Diet Meal Plans

Each stage of the diet offers you three different eating plans.

You may want to follow the Summary Plans, which give you the
general types and exact amounts of foods to eat. With this diet, use
the exchange (or equivalency) tables included in the chapter. The
exchange tables list the foods that are essentially the same in calorie
content as other foods. For example, let's say the menu calls for ½
cup cooked vegetables. Just look at the exchange table for vegetables
to see which ones you can choose from. On that table, you'll notice
that 6 ounces of tomato juice is the same as ½ cup of cooked
vegetables. This means you can have the juice in place of the vegetable
—but only if you have 6 ounces, not 8 or 10 ounces.

You may want to follow the Standard Diet, which gives you two
weeks of simple yet appetizing meals. (If you follow this diet for four
weeks, simply repeat the two weeks.)

If you truly love to cook (and eat), try the Chef's Menu, two
weeks of meals that come straight from some of the finest professional

cooks in Paris. (Again, if you follow this diet for four weeks, repeat the two weeks.)

Finally, you could combine the three plans. For example, you might follow the Summary Plan for busy days; the Standard Diet for evening meals or restful days; and the Chef's Menu for weekends or whenever you want gourmet meals that are quick and easy to prepare. We have also included some suggestions for light meals to take with you to work.

If you don't like a meal on either the Standard Diet or Chef's Menu, that's fine, too. Follow the Summary Plan guidelines, and create your own substitute meal. Just don't eat more than what is allowed in the summary guidelines.

You can also move some foods from one meal to another. Instead of drinking a glass of juice at breakfast, have it at lunch or save a piece of fruit from lunch and eat it as a snack after dinner. Just don't have the food twice. However, don't move protein-rich foods such as meat, fish, or eggs from one meal to another; keep them where they are. You can see which foods are high in protein by checking the protein exchange lists.

If you find other tips that work for you, please let us know. Write to us at

P.O Box 33-1054
Miami, FL 33233-1054

People all over the world are following the program, and we're always looking for ways to make it even easier.

Now, it's time to start the Paris Diet. We've designed it so that you can succeed—you're going to lose weight, and you're going to keep it off. Painlessly, tastefully, and best of all—for good!

PART TWO

⸻ ❧ ⸻

The Paris Diet: The Preparation Program

STAGE ONE   *(2–4 weeks)*
STAGE TWO   *(2–4 weeks)*

CHAPTER 5

---◆---

The Preparation Program:
Stage One

*W*elcome to the beginning of the Paris Diet—the Preparation Program. This is the first stop for anyone who:

was on a diet less than two months ago or
always eats very little

If you fit this description, you are what we call a "life-dieter." As explained in Chapter 2, your body has become so efficient that it is hard for you to lose weight on any plan, unless you literally starve yourself (not a wise idea—you can damage your health). You are the person for whom the Paris Diet was originally designed.

By following the 1,200 calorie plan and then the 1,400 calorie plan for two weeks each, your body will be trained to accept a normal caloric intake. This will prepare it for the Weight Loss Program.

Don't think that you're marking time during this stage and that the "real" diet comes later. Even though you'll be eating more, you may lose a few pounds because this program is high in protein. High protein diets help you to lose weight because:

• you lose fat, not muscle. Some very low-calorie diets result in muscle loss, which leaves you feeling weak and dizzy, and they can even be dangerous;
• protein helps eliminate the hunger pangs that often plague dieters and ultimately cause a diet to fail;
• your metabolism burns more calories to transform protein into a form it can use than it does with carbohydrate or fat;
• the body uses fewer calories from protein-rich foods than from foods rich in carbohydrate or fat because it becomes less efficient and burns off the extra calories as heat.

If you are a heavy eater (usually men), are significantly overweight, and/or rarely diet, skip this stage and move right to the Weight Loss or Adjustment Programs (see Chapter 3).

There are a Few Things You Should Know Before Starting.

1. Use the general tips in Chapter 4.

2. Although the Weight Loss Program eliminates all fat from your meals, you can have some during the Preparation Program, but it is restricted. Use no more than one pat of butter or margarine, and no more than 1 tablespoon of oil or regular salad dressing each day.

3. Exercise can and should be normal, without being overly strenuous. See Chapter 12 for our program.

4. You'll be eating cottage cheese and yogurt, so remember to prepare it in tasty low-calorie ways. You can eat it plain (without sugar, but artificial sweeteners are permitted), or you can add your daily allowance of chopped or puréed fruit. You can also make it a savory treat by adding pepper, herbs, or spices.

5. Instead of regular salad dressing or oil, try our special dressings and sauces for maximum flavor on salads and foods. A light dressing/ sauce can be made from lemon juice, herbs, pepper, vinegar, and a small chopped onion (approximately 5 calories per tablespoon). Sauces can be made from vegetable purées. Reduce tomatoes, eggplants, mushrooms, watercress, celery, leeks, and/or diced carrots to a pulp through long, slow cooking; add spices and herbs; then use them to season dishes (about 5 calories per tablespoon). You can also use the following recipes (page numbers are in parentheses):

FOR SALADS

Sauce Verte/Green Dressing (page 252)

Sauce Menthe/Mint Vinegar (page 248)

Sauce Sontay/Creamy Spinach Dressing (page 249)

Sauce Yogourt/Yogurt Sauce (page 249)

Sauce Tomates aux Aromates/Spicy Tomato Sauce (page 253)

Vinaigre Zéro/Red Vinaigrette (page 247)

Sauce Roquefort/Roquefort Cheese Dressing (page 252)

Sauce Grande Bêche/Watercress Dressing (page 250)

FOR SALADS, POULTRY, VEAL, AND BOILED FISH
Sauce Aïoli/Creamed Garlic Dressing (page 250)

FOR SALADS, POULTRY, AND VEAL
Sauce Provençale/Vinaigrette with Tarragon (page 248)

FOR VEGETABLES AND FISH
Sauce Maraîchère/Tomato and Lemon Sauce with Herbs (page 253)

FOR ZUCCHINI, COLD MEAT, AND FISH
Sauce Tomates à la Chinoise/Chinese-Style Tomato Sauce (page 254)

FOR EGGPLANT, ZUCCHINI, AND PASTA
Sauce Saint-Jeannet/Piperade Dressing (page 251)

6. Check the following lists of prohibited and authorized foods. You will see that on Stage One only bread is permitted in the starch category; on Stage Two, all starches are allowed.

The Preparation Program

Prohibited Foods

For easier selection, here is a list of foods you cannot eat during the Preparation Program. Despite the restrictions, you can still have great meals. Our special dressings and sauces can make most foods taste delicious and satisfying. If you try some of our recipes, you can be eating dishes and desserts like Tarragon-Flavored Chicken, Fresh Salmon Steamed with Vegetables, Frozen Yogurt with Kiwi Sauce, and Strawberries in Champagne.

A prohibited food will occasionally be included in the meal plans, however, to give your mind and taste buds a treat, but don't add one yourself. Follow the meal plans carefully, and only add indulgences where indicated.

SUGAR AND SWEETENED PRODUCTS
sugar, honey, jams, "diet jams," jellies, cookies, pastries, ice cream, sherbet, candies, chocolate, chocolate-flavored drinks, chewing gum with sugar, sorbitol or xylitol (sweeteners that contain significant calories), yogurt or other dairy products with flavorings or fruit

added, candied fruit, fruit in syrup, canned fruit compote, dried fruits (apricots, dates, figs, prunes, raisins, etc.), syrups, canned or bottled fruit juices, soda, cereal bars

STARCHES
Stage One: flaky rolls, crackers, melba toast, breadsticks, matzo, cocktail snack crackers, cereals, pasta, rice, semolina, potatoes, dried legumes (white beans, lentils, split peas, chick peas)
Stage Two: NO STARCHES ARE PROHIBITED

ALCOHOL
all, including flambéed meats, wine sauces, etc.

FATTY FOODS
sauces, fried foods, French fries, potato chips, doughnuts, pizza, quiche, avocados, and anything cooked with oil or fat
Deli Meats: pâté, salami, bologna, frankfurters, sausages, wursts, corned beef, pastrami, tongue
Fatty Meats: pork, mutton, lamb, duck, goose, venison, fatty cuts of beef (like filet mignon or chuck)
Fish and Shellfish: eel, lamprey, breaded fish, fish canned in oil, clams, oysters
Dairy Foods with high fat content: cheeses with greater than 50 percent fat content: Roquefort, Gorgonzola, bleu, Brillat-Savarin, St. Andre, Boursault, Caprice des Dieux, regular and goat cheeses with boosted cream content, creamed cheese, creamed Swiss cheese; regular or creamed cottage cheese or yogurt, whole milk
Nuts: all, including almonds, peanuts, hazelnuts, walnuts, cashews, pine nuts, Brazils

Authorized Foods

Here are the foods you can eat. If you think the prohibited list cut out all delightful foods, think again. There's plenty left, and all of it healthy for mind, body, and figure. Try our special sauces and dressings to add bulk and flavoring to any meal. Shrimp Parfaits, Zucchini with Meat Stuffing, and Baked Apple Surprise are just some of the dishes you and your family can enjoy on this stage of the program.

LEAN, TRIMMED MEATS

beef, veal, chicken (all poultry to be eaten without skin), pheasant, turkey and chicken cutlets, roast turkey, rabbit, lean lamb; very lean roast pork, filet of pork or pork chop can be eaten once a week

LEAN FISH

cod, haddock, pollack, lemon sole, sole, bass, whiting, ray, red mullet, red snapper, turbot

FATTY FISH

shad, anchovies, carp, herring, lake trout, mackerel, sardines, salmon, tuna, all packed in water (no oil)

EAT FISH, LEAN OR FATTY, SEVERAL TIMES EACH WEEK

FRESH FRUITS AND VEGETABLES

STARCHES

Stage One: breads (white or whole wheat, no fruit or honey added)
Stage Two: flaky rolls, crackers, melba toast, breadsticks, matzo, cocktail snack crackers, cereals, pasta, rice, semolina, potatoes, dried legumes (white beans, lentils, split peas, chick peas)

DAIRY FOODS

cheeses with less than 50 percent fat content: low-fat Camembert, Comte, Coulommiers, low-fat Brie, Gruyère, Port du Salut, Edam, Gouda, Mimolette, Cheshire, low-fat goat cheese, Roblochon, Saint-Nectaire, Tomme; 1-2 percent low-fat plain yogurt, low-fat plain cottage cheese

Now you're ready to start. The Paris Diet offers you three menu choices for Stage One (1,200 calories) and Stage Two (1,400 calories) of the Preparation Program. You can follow the Summary Plan, which tells you the basic foods and amounts you have to eat. Use the following exchange (equivalency) tables. They list foods which are the exact equivalents in calorie content of others.

You might follow the Standard Diet, which gives you two weeks of simple, yet appetizing meals. If you love fine food, try our Chef's Menu, which comes from some of the finest professional cooks in Paris!

Finally, you could combine them. For example, you might follow the Summary Plan for busy days or at a restaurant; the Standard Diet for evening meals or lazy days around the house; and the Chef's Menu for weekends or whenever you want gourmet meals that are quick and easy to prepare.

The Preparation Program: Exchange (Equivalency) Tables

The following tables list foods in different categories that are approximately the same, calorie-wise, as other foods. You should use them in two ways. First, these tables will form the basis of the Summary Plan. If lunch calls for ½ cup of cooked vegetables, just look at the vegetable exchange list to see which ones you can choose from.

You can also use these lists to vary your diet if you are following the set menu plans. This is advisable since boredom sabotages any regimen. Simply pick a food from the lists that equals the one in the plan and substitute it. Make sure you use the quantity listed or it won't be equal in caloric value to the food for which it's being exchanged. For example, if you don't feel like having ½ cup of beets, exchange it for 6 ounces of tomato juice—not 4 or 8 ounces but 6 ounces.

Not all foods in the menu plans will have exchanges.

Each one of the foods contained within a numbered list is equal to all others in that list. You can also choose to make two exchanges: For instance, if you want to eat 1 apple, you can either exchange it for 1 small banana, or for 10 cherries plus ½ cup of orange juice. It's up to you.

If the menu calls for 4 ounces of beef, and the exchange table lists beef in quantities of 1 ounce, remember to multiply all the other quantities in the list by 4 if you are exchanging for the beef. In other words, since 1 ounce of beef equals 1 slice of low-fat cheese, 4 ounces of beef would be equal to 4 slices of low-fat cheese.

I. Vegetable Exchanges (for ½ cup cooked or 1 cup raw)

asparagus
beans (green or wax)
bean sprouts
beets
broccoli
Brussels sprouts
cabbage (all kinds)
carrots
catsup, 2 tablespoons
cauliflower
celery
cucumber

eggplant
leafy greens (all kinds)
mushrooms
okra
onion
pepper (red or green)
rutabaga
sauerkraut
squash, summer
tomato
tomato or vegetable juice,
   6 ounces

II. Fruit Exchanges

FRUITS

apple, ½ medium
applesauce, ½ cup
apricots, dried, 4 halves
apricots, fresh, 2 medium
banana, ½ small
blueberries, ½ cup
cantaloupe (6-inch diameter),
   ¼ medium
cherries, 10 large
dates, 2
figs, dried, 1 small
fruit cocktail, canned, ½ cup
grapefruit, ½ small
grapes, 15 small

JUICES

apple, pineapple
grapefruit, orange, ½ cup

honeydew melon (7-inch
   diameter), ⅓
mango, ½ small
nectarine, 1 small
orange, 1 small
papaya, ⅓ medium
peach, 1 medium
pear, 1 small
pineapple, ½ cup
prunes, dried, 2
raisins, 2 tablespoons
strawberries, ¾ cup
tangerine, 1 large
watermelon, 1 cup cubed

grape, prune, ¼ cup

III. Starch Exchanges (cooked servings)

BREADS

bagel, ½

bun for hamburger or
  hot dog, ½

cornbread (1½-inch diameter),
  1 cube

dinner roll (2-inch diameter), 1

English muffin, ½

plain bread (no honey or fruit
  added), 1 slice

tortilla (6-inch diameter), 1

CRACKERS

graham (2½-inch square), 2

matzo (4 by 6 inches), ½

melba toast, 4

oyster crackers (½ cup), 20

pretzels, 8 rings

rye krisps, 3

saltines, 5

CEREALS

bran, 5 tablespoons

dry flakes, ⅔ cup

dry puffed, 1½ cups

hot cereal such as oatmeal,
  farina, ½ cup

pastas, ½ cup

rice, ½ cup

wheat germ, 2 tablespoons

STARCHY VEGETABLES

beans or peas (plain),
  ½ cup

corn, ⅓ cup or ½ medium ear

parsnips, ⅔ cup

potatoes, white, 1 small or
  ½ cup

potatoes, sweet or yams, ¼ cup

pumpkin, ¾ cup

squash, winter, ½ cup

DESSERTS

angel cake, 1½ inch square

fat-free sherbet, 4 ounces

IV. Protein Exchanges (cooked weight)

beef, dried, chipped, 1 ounce

beef, lamb, pork, veal (lean
  only), 1 ounce

cheese, hard, ½ ounce

cheese, low fat, 1 ounce or
  1 slice

fish, 1 ounce

lobster, 1 small tail

oysters, clams, shrimps,
  5 medium

peanut butter, 2 teaspoons

poultry, without skin, 1 ounce

cottage cheese, plain, low fat,
 ¼ cup *
egg, 1 medium

salmon, pink, canned, ¼ cup
tuna, packed in water, ¼ cup

V. Dairy Exchanges
cheese, hard, ½ ounce
cheese, low fat, 1 ounce or
 1 slice
cottage cheese, plain, low fat,
 ¼ cup

milk, 1% fat, ½ cup
milk, skim, ⅔ cup
yogurt, plain, low fat, ½ cup

VI. Fat Exchanges
avocado (4-inch diameter), ⅛
bacon, crisp, 1 slice
butter or margarine, 1 pat
French dressing, 1 tablespoon
mayonnaise, 2 teaspoons
oil, 2 teaspoons (all kinds)

olives, 5 small
peanuts, 10
Roquefort dressing, 1 tablespoon
Thousand Island dressing,
 1 tablespoon
walnuts, 6 small

The Preparation Program: Stage One
Summary for Easy Reference

On this stage of the diet, you will eat certain basic foods each day. If you don't want to follow the Standard Diet or Chef's Menu, use this summary for any or all of the days. You might choose to follow the Chef's Menu on the weekends, but on a busy Monday, substitute the simple foods listed below.

If you want to have even more choice in the selection of your daily meals, refer to the exchange tables to find out which foods are the exact equivalents of the ones below. If you do make a substitution, use the exact quantities in the tables. For example, 1 cup of plain low-fat yogurt is equal to 1⅓ cups of skim milk. You could have either and adhere to the diet. However, if you drink 2 cups of skim

---

* Note: Cheeses contain good amounts of protein and calcium; therefore, they are listed in two tables and can be used either as an exchange for a protein-rich food or as an exchange for a dairy food.

milk in place of 1 cup of yogurt, you'd be consuming too many calories.

You might want to photocopy the summary page to have with you when you're away from home, so you'll never doubt how much and what to eat.

The Preparation Program: Stage One

Summary Plan

BREAKFAST

½ cup plain, low-fat yogurt
2 slices of bread (any type of regular white or whole wheat
    with no fruit or honey added)
½ cup fruit juice (if you eliminate one fruit serving
    from another meal)
1 pat butter or margarine
beverage

LUNCH

small green salad or 3 oz raw vegetables with light dressing
4 oz lean meat or skinless poultry or fish, cooked without fat
¾ cup boiled or steamed vegetables, cooked without fat
1 slice or 1 oz low-fat cheese
1 medium-size piece or ½ cup fruit
beverage

DINNER

4 oz lean meat or skinless poultry or fish, cooked without fat
¾ cup boiled or steamed vegetables, cooked without fat
½ cup plain low-fat yogurt
1 medium-size piece or ½ cup fruit
beverage

For Men

Since men have more muscle mass and therefore slightly higher protein needs than women, men must add one of the following:

2 whites of eggs (no yolks), hard boiled, chopped into salads, or
¼ cup low-fat cottage cheese, or
½ cup plain low-fat yogurt, or
1 slice of ham or turkey or roast beef

These extra foods can be eaten at any point in the day and should be added to the Summary Plan, Standard Diet, and Chef's Menu.

The Preparation Program: Stage One
Cold Meals You Can Take to Work

With our busy schedule, many of us don't have the time to prepare elaborate lunches or go out to restaurants. Therefore, the following are some examples of cold meals for lunch or early dinner that you may easily prepare at home and take to the office. By following the Summary Plan, you may also come up with your own ideas for simple bagable items—just make sure you stick to the basic guidelines.

MEAL #1
small raw vegetable salad with 1
    tbs light dressing
1 roast chicken leg or 4 oz white
    meat chicken
1 slice or 1 oz low-fat cheese
1 pear or fruit equivalent
beverage

MEAL #2
1 cup low-fat cottage cheese
    with 1 piece chopped fruit
2 slices bread with 1 pat butter
    or margarine
beverage

MEAL #3
medium mixed salad (diced hard
    cheese, small dices of ham,
    and a few flakes of plain tuna
    fish) with 1 tbs light dressing
½ cup plain low-fat yogurt
1 fruit
beverage

MEAL #4
medium bowl sliced cucumber
    salad with 1 tbs light dressing
sandwich of 1 slice cold lean
    meat, 1 slice or 1 oz low-fat
    cheese, and 2 slices bread
    with 1 pat butter or
    margarine
1 fruit
beverage

(You might also want to pack any cold meals from the Standard Diet or the Chef's Menu, and any hot meals if there's a microwave at work.)

The Preparation Program: Stage One

The Standard Diet

The following menu plans are for two weeks of the 1,200-calorie Standard Diet, which you should find tasty and satisfying. All foods are simple to find and prepare. However, if you want to add a little gourmet flavor, we have included some quick and easy recipes you can substitute in place of the regular meals. These recipes can be found on the pages listed in the menu plans.

DAY ONE

BREAKFAST
½ cup plain low-fat yogurt
½ cup orange juice
2 slices any type of bread (toast)
  with 1 pat butter or
  margarine
beverage

LUNCH
small green salad with 1 tbs light
  dressing
4 oz sole or other white fish
¾ cup cooked spinach,
  tomatoes, or broccoli
1 slice or 1 oz low-fat cheese
beverage

DINNER
4 oz lean beef
¾ cup cooked summer squash,
  mixed vegetables, or turnips
½ cup plain low-fat yogurt
1 piece fruit
beverage

DAY TWO

BREAKFAST
2 slices bread (toast) with 1 pat
    butter or margarine
2 slices or 2 oz low-fat cheese
½ cup grapefruit juice
beverage

LUNCH
4 oz grilled lean steak
¾ cup cooked green beans,
    mixed vegetables, or zucchini
1 cup plain low-fat yogurt
beverage

DINNER
small mixed salad with 1 tbs
    light dressing
4 oz roast chicken
¾ cup cooked peas, carrots, or
    cauliflower
½ cup low-fat cottage cheese
medium baked apple
beverage

DAY THREE

BREAKFAST
1 cup any unsweetened cereal
    with ½ cup skim milk, no
    sugar, artificial sweetener
    permitted
½ cup grapefruit juice
beverage

LUNCH
¾ cup cooked carrots, green
    beans, or spinach with 1 pat
    butter or margarine
2 eggs, any style
1 slice or 1 oz low-fat cheese
beverage

DINNER
medium bowl vegetable soup
4 oz lean veal
½ cup stewed tomatoes,
    Brussels sprouts, or
    8 asparagus spears
¾ cup low-fat cottage cheese
    with 1 piece of chopped fruit
beverage

DAY FOUR

BREAKFAST
1 English muffin with 1 pat
    butter or margarine
1 slice or 1 oz low-fat cheese
½ cup orange juice
beverage

LUNCH
large mixed salad with 1 tbs
    light dressing
4 oz lean hamburger
½ cup low-fat cottage cheese
beverage

DINNER
4 oz grilled fish, any kind
½ cup cooked zucchini or
    mushrooms
1 cup plain low-fat yogurt with
    1 piece chopped fruit
beverage

DAY FIVE

BREAKFAST
1 cup any unsweetened cereal
    with ½ cup skim milk, no
    sugar, artificial sweetener
    permitted
½ cup orange juice
beverage

LUNCH
large mixed salad with 1 tbs
    light dressing
4 oz lean beef or grilled shrimp
2 slices or 2 oz low-fat cheese
beverage

DINNER
medium spinach salad with 1 tbs
    light dressing
4 oz turkey or chicken breast
¾ cup cooked cabbage,
    broccoli, or carrots with 1 pat
    butter or margarine
½ cup plain low-fat yogurt with
    1 piece chopped fruit
beverage

DAY SIX

BREAKFAST

2 slices bread (toast) with 1 pat
    butter or margarine
½ cup plain low-fat yogurt with
    1 piece chopped fruit
beverage

LUNCH

small green salad with 1 tbs light
    dressing
4 oz roast chicken
¾ cup cooked carrots or
    broccoli (or *Carottes Vichy*/
    Sliced Carrots with Parsley,
    page 257)
½ cup plain low-fat yogurt
beverage

DINNER

6 oz tomato or vegetable juice
small mixed salad with 1 tbs
    light dressing
4 oz salmon or trout
1 oz low-fat cheese
1 apple or pear or peach
beverage

DAY SEVEN

BREAKFAST

1 cup any unsweetened cereal
    with ½ cup skim milk, no
    sugar, artificial sweetener
    permitted
½ cup grapefruit juice
beverage

LUNCH

tomato salad (1 medium sliced
    tomato with 1 tbs light
    dressing)
4 oz lean hamburger with 1 slice
    cheese (or *Filets de Boeuf aux
    Échalotes*/Beef Filets with
    Shallots, page 267)
beverage

DINNER

medium chef's salad with 2 oz
    turkey, 2 oz roast beef, 1 oz
    low-fat cheese, tomato,
    lettuce, and 1 tbs light

DINNER (cont'd)
  dressing (or *Courgettes Farcies/*
  Stuffed Zucchini, page 260)
  ½ cup plain low-fat yogurt
  1 piece fruit
  beverage

DAY EIGHT

BREAKFAST
1 English muffin with 1 pat
  butter or margarine
½ cup plain low-fat yogurt
1 apple or orange or 15 grapes
beverage

LUNCH
medium mixed salad with 1 oz
  diced or sliced low-fat cheese
  and 1 tbs light dressing
4 oz lean ham
½ cup plain low-fat yogurt with
  1 piece chopped fruit
beverage

DINNER
6 oz tomato or vegetable juice
4 oz chicken or turkey (or *Poulet
  en Croûte de Sel*/Chicken Baked
  in a Salt Crust, page 281)
¾ cup cooked zucchini, carrots,
  or broccoli
beverage

DAY NINE

BREAKFAST
1 cup any unsweetened cereal
  with ½ cup skim milk, no
  sugar, artificial sweetener
  permitted
½ cup plain low-fat yogurt
½ cup orange juice
beverage

LUNCH
large mixed salad with 1 tbs
  light dressing, with 2 eggs any
  style (or *Piperade*/Scrambled
  Eggs with Tomatoes and
  Sweet Peppers, page 286)
1 slice or 1 oz low-fat cheese
beverage

DINNER
small green salad with lemon
  juice
4 oz broiled salmon or trout
¾ cup cooked tomatoes or
  carrots
½ cup plain low-fat yogurt with
  1 piece chopped fruit
beverage

DAY TEN

BREAKFAST
2 slices bread (toast) with 1 pat
  butter or margarine
½ cup plain low-fat yogurt
beverage

LUNCH
medium mixed salad with 1 oz
  diced low-fat cheese and
  1 tbs light dressing (or
  Ratatouille/Stewed Vegetables
  Mediterranean Style,
  page 263)
4 oz roast chicken
¾ cup cooked green beans,
  squash, or Brussels sprouts
1 piece fruit
beverage

DINNER
small bowl vegetable soup
4 oz lean steak
½ cup cooked peppers, Brussels
  sprouts, or stewed tomatoes
1 cup plain low-fat yogurt
1 pear or apple or 15 grapes
beverage

DAY ELEVEN

BREAKFAST
1 English muffin with 1 pat
   butter or margarine
1 slice or 1 oz low-fat cheese
½ cup unsweetened grapefruit
   juice
beverage

LUNCH
medium mixed salad with 1 tbs
   light dressing
4 oz sliced turkey or chicken
½ cup plain low-fat yogurt with
   1 piece chopped fruit
beverage

DINNER
small mixed salad with 1 tbs
   light dressing
4 oz broiled lean steak
½ cup cooked mixed vegetables,
   green beans, or cauliflower
½ cup low-fat cottage cheese
   with ½ cup fruit canned in
   its own juice
beverage

DAY TWELVE

BREAKFAST
2 slices bread (toast) with 1 pat
   butter or margarine
1 egg, any style
beverage

LUNCH
medium green salad with 1 tbs
   light dressing
3 oz lean steak (or *Filets de Boeuf
   aux Échalotes*/Beef Filets with
   Shallots, page 267)
½ cup lemon sherbet with
   artificial sweetener or piece of
   fruit
beverage

DINNER
6 oz tomato or vegetable juice
   (or *Aspic de Légumes au Coulis
   de Tomates*/Vegetable Aspic

with Tomato Sauce,
    page 264)
3 oz trout, sole, or snapper
¾ cup cooked mixed vegetables,
    broccoli, or green beans
    topped with 1 oz grated low-
    fat cheese
1 cup plain low-fat yogurt with
    1 piece chopped fruit
beverage

DAY THIRTEEN

BREAKFAST
½ cup plain low-fat yogurt
1 slice bread (any type) with
    1 pat butter or margarine
½ cup orange juice
beverage

LUNCH
medium green salad with 1 oz
    diced low-fat cheese and
    1 tbs light dressing
3–4 oz individual can of water-
    packed tuna or salmon
2 crackers
beverage

DINNER
small mixed salad with 1 tbs
    light dressing
4 oz lean pork with ¾ cup
    baked tomato, cauliflower, or
    brussels sprouts (or *Porc
    Colombo*/Pork Tenderloin with
    Eggplant, page 271)
½ cup plain low-fat yogurt with
    1 piece chopped fruit
beverage

DAY FOURTEEN

BREAKFAST
2 slices bread (toast) with 1 pat
  butter or margarine
½ cup plain low-fat yogurt
½ cup unsweetened orange
  juice
beverage

LUNCH
large spinach salad with 1 tbs
  light dressing
4 oz cold chicken or turkey
beverage

DINNER
small mixed salad with 1 tbs
  light dressing
4 oz lean lamb or beef
¾ cup steamed zucchini,
  broccoli, or eggplant, topped
  with 1 oz grated low-fat
  cheese
½ cup plain low-fat yogurt with
  1 piece chopped fruit
beverage

The Preparation Program: Stage One

Chef's Menu

If you love great food but need to follow a structured diet, you've just found the ultimate solution. Here is a true gourmet's delight— our Chef's Menu, from some of the greatest cooks in Paris. Although these recipes (listed by page number) are easy to prepare, they are no less delightful than the finest meals served along the banks of the Seine.

DAY ONE

BREAKFAST

2 slices bread (toast) with 1 pat
    butter or margarine
½ cup plain low-fat yogurt
½ cup orange juice
beverage

LUNCH

*Gâteau de Carottes au Coulis
    d'Asperges* (Carrot Cakes with
    Asparagus Sauce), page 258
Fondant de Volaille au Whisky
    (Chicken Salad with Whiskey
    Dressing), page 282
½ cup plain low-fat yogurt
1 apple
beverage

DINNER

small green salad with 1 tbs light
    dressing
Coquilles St. Jacques à la Provençale
    (Scallops à la Provençale),
    page 296
1 slice or 1 oz low-fat cheese
beverage

DAY TWO

BREAKFAST

1 cup any unsweetened cereal
    with ½ cup skim milk, no
    sugar, artificial sweetener
    permitted
½ cup grapefruit juice
beverage

LUNCH

small *salade vermeil* (salad of
    radishes, mushrooms, and
    lemon juice)
Saumon Cuit à Basse Température
    (Salmon Cooked at Low
    Temperature), page 292
½ cup plain low-fat yogurt
beverage

DINNER
Salade Marignan (Mixed Vegetable
   Salad), page 245
Omelette Soufflée (Fluffy Omelet),
   page 288
1 slice or 1 oz low-fat cheese
½ cup mixed fruit salad
beverage

DAY THREE

BREAKFAST
2 slices bread (toast) with 1 pat
   butter or margarine
1 slice or 1 oz low-fat cheese
beverage

LUNCH
*Méli-Mélo de Crevettes Roses aux
   Huîtres* (Hodgepodge of Pink
   Shrimp with Oysters),
   page 298
Filet de Boeuf Grand-Mère (Old-
   Fashioned Filet of Beef),
   page 265
½ cup plain low-fat yogurt
salad of ½ cup oranges (fresh or
   canned in their own juice, not
   sweetened), with fresh mint
beverage

DINNER
small bowl vegetable soup
*Pilon de Volaille Cuit aux Senteurs
   d'Estragon* (Tarragon-Flavored
   Chicken), page 276
½ cup low-fat cottage cheese
   with 1 piece chopped fruit
beverage

DAY FOUR

BREAKFAST
2 slices bread (toast) with 1 pat
butter or margarine
½ cup plain low-fat yogurt
1 orange
beverage

LUNCH
Salade de Haricots Verts Printanière
(Springtime Green Bean
Salad), page 246
*Gratin de St. Jacques à l'Effiloché
d'Endives* (Scallops Gratin with
a Fringe of Endives),
page 294
1 slice or 1 oz low-fat cheese
beverage

DINNER
small green salad with 1 tbs light
dressing
*Croquette d'Agneau en Bouquet de
Légumes* (Lamb with Mixed
Végetables), page 270
Yogourt Glacé au Coulis de Kiwi
(Frozen Yogurt with Kiwi
Sauce), page 313
beverage

DAY FIVE

BREAKFAST
2 slices bread (toast) with 1 pat
butter or margarine
1 soft-boiled egg
1 slice or 1 oz low-fat cheese
beverage

LUNCH
1 oz low-fat white cheese with
6 cucumber slices and chives
Filet de Dinde en Habit-Vert
(Turkey Filet in French
Academy Costume),
page 284
½ cup fresh pineapple chunks
beverage

DINNER
Gaspacho de Tomates (Tomato
     Gazpacho), page 243
Courgettes Farçies à la Viande
     (Zucchini with Meat Stuffing),
     page 261
½ cup stewed apples and pears
beverage

DAY SIX

BREAKFAST
1 cup any unsweetened cereal
     with ½ cup skim milk, no
     sugar, artificial sweetener
     permitted
½ cup mixed fruit salad
beverage

LUNCH
Soufflé de Brocolis aux Deux Épices
     (Broccoli Soufflé with Two
     Spices), page 256
Parfait de Gambas (Shrimp
     Parfaits), page 297
½ cup purée of celery
1 fruit
beverage

DINNER
small raw mushroom salad with
     lemon juice
Sauté de Veau aux Petits Légumes
     (Sautéed Veal with
     Vegetables), page 268
1 slice or 1 oz low-fat cheese
     with 2 crackers
beverage

DAY SEVEN

BREAKFAST
2 slices bread (toast) with 1 pat
   butter or margarine
½ cup plain low-fat yogurt
beverage

LUNCH
small green salad with 1 tbs light
   dressing
*Jambonnette de Volaille au Parfum de
   Truffes* (Chicken Flavored with
   Truffles), page 275
1 slice or 1 oz low-fat cheese
Soupe de Fraises au Champagne
   (Strawberries in Champagne),
   page 312
beverage

DINNER
½ pink grapefruit, without
   sugar
Petit Rouget au Fenouil Frais (Red
   Mullet or Snapper with Fresh
   Fennel), page 300
½ cup plain low-fat yogurt
beverage

DAY EIGHT

BREAKFAST
½ cup cooked farina or any
   unsweetened cereal with
   ½ cup skim milk, no sugar,
   artificial sweetener permitted
½ cup grapefruit juice
beverage

LUNCH
small mixed salad (lettuce,
   tomatoes, carrots) with 1 tbs
   light dressing
*Blanc de Volaille aux Spaghetti de
   Concombre* (Chicken Breasts
   with Cucumber Spaghetti),
   page 273
1 slice or 1 oz low-fat cheese
beverage

DINNER
small bowl vegetable soup
Rôti de Bar au Varech (Broiled
   Bass with Seaweed),
   page 289
½ cup plain low-fat yogurt
Brochettes de Fruits en Papillotes
   (Fruit Skewers), page 316
beverage

DAY NINE

BREAKFAST
2 slices bread (toast) with 1 pat
   butter or margarine
1 slice or 1 oz low-fat cheese
beverage

LUNCH
small bowl of carrot and
   cucumber sticks, raw
   cauliflowerets with 1 tbs light
   dressing
Coeur de Filet de Boeuf aux Épices
   (Beef Filet with Spices),
   page 266
Pétales de Kiwi au Jus de Fraises
   (Kiwi Petals with Strawberry
   Purée), page 313
beverage

DINNER
Asperges aux Champignons en Duo
   (Duet of Asparagus and
   Mushrooms), page 255
*Petite Nage aux Senteurs d'Herbe
   Folle* (Mixed Seafood Flavored
   with Wild Herbs), page 308
1 mango or 1 apple
beverage

DAY TEN

BREAKFAST
2 slices bread (toast) with 1 pat
   butter or margarine
½ cup plain low-fat yogurt
½ cup orange juice
beverage

LUNCH
Émincé de Volaille aux Deux Choux
   (Chicken Breasts with
   Broccoli and Cauliflower),
   page 274
½ cup plain low-fat yogurt
beverage

DINNER
small green salad with 3 oz
   warmed chicken livers and
   sherry vinegar
1 slice or 1 oz low-fat cheese
Pommes Surprises au Four (Baked
   Apple Surprise), page 310
beverage

DAY ELEVEN

BREAKFAST
1 cup any unsweetened cereal
   with ½ cup skim milk, no
   sugar, artificial sweetener
   permitted
beverage

LUNCH
small mixed raw vegetable salad
   with lemon juice and vinegar
Truite au Sel (Trout in Salt),
   page 304
Mousse aux Deux Fruits (Two-Fruit
   Mousse), page 314
beverage

DINNER
steamed leeks or small green
   salad with vinaigrette dressing
*Oeufs Durs ou Pochés Florentine aux
   Épinards* (Hard-Cooked or
   Poached Eggs with Spinach),
   page 287
1 slice or 1 oz low-fat cheese
1 pear
beverage

DAY TWELVE

BREAKFAST
2 slices bread (toast) with 1 pat
    butter or margarine
½ cup plain low-fat yogurt
1 piece fruit
beverage

LUNCH
Courgettes aux Crevettes Roses
    (Zucchini with Pink Shrimp),
    page 262
4 oz broiled steak with mustard
1 slice or 1 oz low-fat cheese
beverage

DINNER
small two-toned salad (carrots
    and white cabbage) with 1 tbs
    light dressing
Suprême de Dinde en Papillotes
    (Turkey Supreme in
    Papillotes), page 285
Gratin de Fraises à la Cannelle
    (Cinnamon-Flavored
    Strawberries), page 312
beverage

DAY THIRTEEN

BREAKFAST
2 slices bread (toast) with 1 pat
    butter or margarine
1 slice or 1 oz low-fat cheese
1 soft-boiled egg
beverage

LUNCH
small green salad with 1 tbs light
    dressing
*Filet de Sole à la Purée de
    Concombre* (Filet of Sole with
    Cucumber Purée), page 301
1 oz low-fat white cheese with
    fresh peach slices
beverage

DINNER
4 oz leg of lamb
½ cup steamed green beans
    with parsley
½ cup plain low-fat yogurt
Aspic de Fruits Frais aux Saveurs
    Exotiques (Fresh Fruit Aspic
    with Exotic Flavors),
    page 315

DAY FOURTEEN

BREAKFAST
rice pudding without sugar,
    sweetened with 2 small
    apricots in their own juice
beverage

LUNCH
small green salad with 1 oz low-
    fat white cheese and 1 tbs
    light dressing
Poulet Pané au Sésame (Breaded
    Chicken with Sesame Seeds),
    page 278
½ cup grilled tomatoes
Mousse au Chocolat Noir Allégé
    (Low-Calorie Dark Chocolate
    Mousse), page 316
beverage

DINNER
1 regular slice melon
St. Pierre au Citron Vert et au Coco
    (Grouper with Lime and
    Coconut), page 290
½ cup steamed zucchini and
    eggplant
½ cup plain low-fat yogurt
beverage

You can follow this menu for only one of the days, on special
occasions, or for the entire two weeks if you really want to eat like
royalty while dieting.

CHAPTER 6

The Preparation Program: Stage Two

*Y*ou have now moved on to Stage Two of the Preparation Program. It is not at all difficult to follow; the only difference between it and Stage One (1,200 calories) is that extra starches have been added, which makes it more similar to your normal diet. Because of the starch, you also get more gourmet recipes from which to choose.

If you are a life-dieter or eat under 1,400 calories daily, you must remain at this stage for an additional two weeks (or better yet, a month) before moving to the Weight Loss Program. Remember to follow all the guidelines on eating and preparation from the previous chapter.

Additional Suggestions for Stage Two

1. If you are taking some of our suggested cold meals to the office, use the Stage One examples (page 75) and get extra starch by adding ⅕ cup of cold cooked rice.

2. On Stage Two, you can have 2 tablespoons of oil or regular salad dressing per day. Better still, in place of regular salad dressing or oil, try our special dressings and sauces for maximum flavor. The lightest dressing/sauce that you can use can be made from lemon juice, herbs, pepper, vinegar, and a small chopped onion (about 5 calories per tablespoon). Sauces can be made from vegetable purées. Reduce tomatoes, eggplants, mushrooms, watercress, celery, leeks, and/or carrots to a pulp through long slow cooking, add spices and herbs, then use to season dishes (about 5 calories per tablespoon). You can also use the following recipes (page numbers are in parentheses):

FOR SALADS
Sauce Verte/Green Dressing (page 252)
Sauce Menthe/Mint Vinegar (page 248)
Sauce Sontay/Creamy Spinach Dressing (page 249)
Sauce Yogourt/Yogurt Sauce (page 249)
Sauce Tomates aux Aromates/Spicy Tomato Sauce (page 253)
Vinaigre Zéro/Red Vinaigrette (page 247)
Sauce Roquefort/Roquefort Cheese Dressing (page 252)
Sauce Grande Bêche/Watercress Dressing (page 250)

FOR SALADS, POULTRY, VEAL, AND BOILED FISH
Sauce Aïoli/Creamed Garlic Dressing (page 250)

FOR SALADS, POULTRY, AND VEAL
Sauce Provençale/Vinaigrette with Tarragon (page 248)

FOR VEGETABLES AND FISH
Sauce Maraîchère/Tomato and Lemon Sauce with Herbs (page 253)

FOR ZUCCHINI, COLD MEAT, AND FISH
Sauce Tomates à la Chinoise/Chinese-Style Tomato Sauce (page 254)

FOR EGGPLANT, ZUCCHINI, AND PASTA
Sauce Saint-Jeannet/Piperade Dressing (page 251)

3. To make starchy foods tastier, season them with 1 tablespoon of our special low-fat sauces or ½ pat of butter or margarine, or 2 tablespoons of grated cheese. But if you do add this extra fat, eliminate the butter or margarine used at breakfast or eliminate 1 tablespoon of regular salad dressing or oil.

The Preparation Program: Stage Two
Summary for Easy Reference

On this stage of the diet, you will eat certain basic foods each day. If you don't want to follow the Standard Diet or Chef's Menu, use this summary for any or all of the days. You might choose to follow the Chef's Menu on the weekends, but on a busy Monday, substitute the simple foods listed below.

If you want to have even more choice in the selection of your daily meals, refer to the exchange tables on page 70 to find out which foods are the exact equivalents of the ones below. If you do make a substitution, use the exact quantities in the tables. For example, 1 cup of plain low-fat yogurt is equal to 1⅓ cups of skim milk. You could have either and adhere to the diet. However, if you drink 2 cups of skim milk in place of the 1 cup of yogurt, you'd be consuming too many calories.

You might want to photocopy the summary page to have with you when you're away from home, so you'll never be in doubt about how much and what to eat.

The Preparation Program: Stage Two
Summary Plan

BREAKFAST

½ cup plain low-fat yogurt or ½ cup low-fat cottage cheese

½ cup unsweetened fruit juice or piece of fruit (can be saved for dessert at lunch or dinner)

2 slices plain bread or toast (any type) with 2 pats butter or margarine

beverage

LUNCH

medium green salad with 1 tbs oil or regular salad dressing

¾ cup cooked or 1½ cups raw vegetables (boiled or steamed without oil or fat)

4 oz meat or fish (cooked without oil or fat—baked, broiled, steamed, or grilled only)

1 oz or 1 slice low-fat cheese

1 slice plain bread or toast (any type) or 4 plain crackers

1 medium-size piece or ½ cup chopped fruit

beverage

DINNER

medium green salad with 1 tbs light dressing

4 oz lean meat or fish (cooked without oil or fat—baked, broiled, steamed or grilled only)

2 medium potatoes or starch equivalents (see exchange tables), cooked without fat

½ cup plain low-fat yogurt or ½ cup low-fat cottage cheese

beverage

For Men

Since men have more muscle mass and therefore slightly higher protein needs than women, men must add one of the following:

2 whites of eggs (no yolks), hard-boiled, chopped into salads, or

¼ cup low-fat cottage cheese, or

½ cup plain low-fat yogurt, or

1 slice of ham or turkey or roast beef

The Preparation Program: Stage Two
The Standard Diet

The following menu plans are for two weeks of the 1,400 calorie Standard Diet. All the foods are simple to find and prepare. If you want to add a little gourmet flavor, we have included some easy recipes to substitute in place of the regular meals. These recipes can be found on the pages listed in menu plans.

DAY ONE

BREAKFAST
½ cup plain low-fat yogurt
½ cup orange juice
2 slices plain bread (any type)
    with 1 pat butter or
    margarine
beverage

LUNCH
medium green salad with 1 tbs
    oil or regular salad dressing
4 oz sole or other white fish
¾ cup cooked spinach,
    tomatoes, or broccoli
1 slice or 1 oz low-fat cheese
1 slice plain bread (any type) or
    4 plain crackers
beverage

DINNER
4 oz lean beef
2 medium potatoes with 1 pat
    butter or margarine
½ cup plain low-fat yogurt
1 piece fruit
beverage

DAY TWO

BREAKFAST
2 slices plain bread (any type)
   with 1 pat butter or
   margarine
2 slices or 2 oz low-fat cheese
½ cup grapefruit juice
beverage

LUNCH
4 oz broiled lean steak
¾ cup cooked green beans,
   mixed vegetables, or zucchini
   with 1 pat butter or
   margarine
½ cup plain low-fat yogurt
1 slice plain bread (any type) or
   4 plain crackers
beverage

DINNER
medium mixed salad with 1 tbs
   oil or regular salad dressing
4 oz roast chicken
1 cup cooked macaroni with
   low-calorie sauce (see our
   recipes)
½ cup low-fat cottage cheese
1 medium baked apple
beverage

DAY THREE

BREAKFAST
1 cup any unsweetened cereal
   with ½ cup skim milk, no
   sugar, artificial sweetener
   permitted
½ cup grapefruit juice
1 slice or 1 oz low-fat cheese
beverage

LUNCH
2 eggs, any style
¾ cup cooked carrots, green
   beans, or spinach with 1 pat
   butter or margarine
1 slice or 1 oz low-fat cheese
1 slice plain bread (any type) or
   4 plain crackers
beverage

DINNER
medium bowl vegetable soup
4 oz lean veal

DINNER (*cont'd*)
⅖ cup cooked rice with 1 pat
    butter or margarine
¾ cup low-fat cottage cheese
    with 1 piece chopped fruit
beverage

DAY FOUR

BREAKFAST
1 English muffin with 1 pat
    butter or margarine
1 slice or 1 oz low-fat cheese
½ cup orange juice
beverage

LUNCH
large mixed salad with 1 tbs oil
    or regular salad dressing
4 oz lean hamburger
½ cup low-fat cottage cheese
1 slice plain bread (any type) or
    4 plain crackers
beverage

DINNER
small green salad with 1 tbs light
    dressing
4 oz broiled fish (any kind)
2 medium potatoes with 1 pat
    butter or margarine
½ cup plain low-fat yogurt with
    1 piece chopped fruit
beverage

DAY FIVE

BREAKFAST
1 cup any unsweetened cereal
    with ½ cup skim milk, no
    sugar, artificial sweetener
    permitted
½ cup orange juice
1 slice or 1 oz low-fat cheese
beverage

LUNCH
large mixed salad with 1 tbs oil
    or regular salad dressing
4 oz lean beef or grilled shrimp
2 slices or 2 oz low-fat cheese
1 slice plain bread (any type) or
    4 plain crackers
beverage

DINNER
medium spinach salad with 1 tbs
    light dressing
4 oz turkey or chicken breast
1½ cup cooked yellow corn
    with 1 pat butter or
    margarine
½ cup plain low-fat yogurt with
    1 piece chopped fruit
beverage

DAY SIX

BREAKFAST
2 slices plain bread (any type)
    with 1 pat butter or
    margarine
½ cup plain low-fat yogurt with
    1 piece chopped fruit
beverage

LUNCH
small green salad with 1 tbs oil
    or regular salad dressing
4 oz roast chicken or chicken
    breast
¾ cup cooked carrots or
    broccoli (or *Carottes Vichy/*
    Sliced Carrots with Parsley,
    page 257)
½ cup plain low-fat yogurt
beverage

DINNER
6 oz tomato or vegetable juice
4 oz salmon or trout
⅘ cup cooked rice with 1 pat
    butter or margarine
1 oz or 1 slice low-fat cheese
1 slice plain bread (any type) or
    4 plain crackers
1 apple or pear or peach
beverage

DAY SEVEN

BREAKFAST
1 cup any unsweetened cereal
   with ½ cup skim milk, no
   sugar, artificial sweetener
   permitted
½ cup grapefruit juice
1 egg, any style
beverage

LUNCH
medium tomato salad with 1 tbs
   oil or regular salad dressing
4 oz lean hamburger with 1 slice
   low-fat cheese (or *Filets de
   Boeuf aux Échalotes*/Beef Filets
   with Shallots, page 267)
beverage

DINNER
large chef's salad with 2 oz
   turkey, 2 oz roast beef, 1 oz
   low-fat cheese, tomato,
   lettuce, and 2 medium boiled,
   chopped potatoes with 1 tbs
   light dressing (or *Courgettes
   Farcies*/Stuffed Zucchini,
   page 260)
½ cup plain low-fat yogurt
1 piece fruit
beverage

DAY EIGHT

BREAKFAST
1 English muffin with 1 pat
   butter or margarine
½ cup plain low-fat yogurt with
   1 piece chopped fruit
beverage

LUNCH
large mixed salad with 1 oz
   diced or sliced low-fat cheese
   and 1 tbs oil or regular salad
   dressing
4 oz lean ham
½ cup plain low-fat yogurt
1 apple or orange or 15 grapes
1 slice plain bread (any type) or
   4 plain crackers
beverage

DINNER

4 oz tomato or vegetable juice
4 oz chicken or turkey (or *Poulet
en Croûte de Sel*/Chicken Baked
in a Salt Crust, page 281)
½ cup cooked zucchini, carrots,
or broccoli
2 medium (1 cup) mashed
potatoes with 1 pat butter or
margarine
beverage

DAY NINE

BREAKFAST

1 cup any unsweetened cereal
with ½ cup skim milk, no
sugar, artificial sweetener
permitted
½ cup plain low-fat yogurt
½ cup orange juice
beverage

LUNCH

large mixed salad with 1 tbs oil
or regular salad dressing plus
2 eggs, any style (or *Piperade/
Scrambled Eggs with
Tomatoes and Sweet Peppers*,
page 286)
1 slice or 1 oz low-fat cheese
1 slice plain bread (any type) or
4 plain crackers
beverage

DINNER

small green salad with 1 tbs light
dressing
4 oz broiled salmon or trout
½ cup cooked tomatoes or
carrots
⅘ cup cooked rice with 1 pat
butter or margarine
½ cup plain low-fat yogurt with
1 piece chopped fruit
beverage

DAY TEN

BREAKFAST
3 slices plain bread (any type)
   with 2 pats butter or
   margarine
½ cup plain low-fat yogurt
beverage

LUNCH
medium mixed salad with 1 oz
   diced or sliced low-fat cheese
   and 1 tbs light dressing (or
   Ratatouille/Stewed Vegetables
   Mediterranean Style,
   page 263)
4 oz roast chicken or chicken
   breast
¾ cup cooked green beans, any
   squash, or Brussels sprouts
1 piece fruit
beverage

DINNER
small bowl vegetable soup
4 oz lean ham
1 cup cooked lentils with 1 pat
   butter or margarine
½ cup plain low-fat yogurt
1 pear or apple or 15 grapes
beverage

DAY ELEVEN

BREAKFAST
1 English muffin with 1 pat
   butter or margarine
1 slice or 1 oz low-fat cheese
½ cup grapefruit juice
beverage

LUNCH
large mixed salad with 1 tbs oil
   or regular salad dressing
4 oz sliced turkey or chicken
½ cup plain low-fat yogurt with
   1 piece chopped fruit
beverage

DINNER
small green salad with 1 tbs light
   dressing
4 oz broiled lean steak

½ cup cooked mixed vegetables,
   green beans, or cauliflower
⅘ cup cooked rice with 1 pat
   butter or margarine
½ cup low-fat cottage cheese
   with ½ piece chopped fruit
beverage

DAY TWELVE

BREAKFAST
2 slices plain bread (any type)
   with 1 pat butter or
   margarine
1 egg, any style
1 slice lean ham
beverage

LUNCH
large green salad with 1 tbs oil
   or regular salad dressing
4 oz lean steak
½ cup lemon sherbet or piece
   of fruit
beverage

DINNER
4 oz tomato or vegetable juice
   (or *Aspic de Légumes au Coulis
   de Tomates*/Vegetable Aspic
   with Tomato Sauce,
   page 264)
4 oz trout, sole, or snapper
½ cup cooked mixed vegetables,
   broccoli, or green beans
2 medium (1 cup) mashed
   potatoes topped with 1 oz
   grated low-fat cheese and
   1 pat butter or margarine
½ cup plain low-fat yogurt with
   1 piece chopped fruit
beverage

DAY THIRTEEN

BREAKFAST
2 slices plain bread (any type)
 with 1 pat butter or
 margarine
½ cup plain low-fat yogurt
½ cup orange juice
beverage

LUNCH
large green salad with 1 oz diced
 or sliced low-fat cheese and
 1 tbs oil or regular salad
 dressing
3–4 oz individual can water-
 packed tuna or salmon
4 crackers
beverage

DINNER
small mixed salad with 1 tbs
 light dressing
4 oz lean pork with ½ cup
 baked tomato and ⅓ cup
 cooked rice with 1 pat butter
 or margarine (or *Porc Colombo/*
 Pork Tenderloin with
 Eggplant, page 271)
½ cup plain low-fat yogurt with
 1 piece chopped fruit
beverage

DAY FOURTEEN

BREAKFAST
2 slices plain bread (any type)
 with 1 pat butter or
 margarine
½ cup plain low-fat yogurt
½ cup orange juice
beverage

LUNCH
large spinach salad with 1 tbs oil
 or regular salad dressing
4 oz cold chicken or turkey
1 slice or 1 oz low-fat cheese
1 piece fruit
beverage

DINNER
large mixed salad with 1 tbs
 light dressing
4 oz lean lamb or beef

⅕ cup red kidney beans with
1 pat butter or margarine
½ cup plain low-fat yogurt
beverage

The Preparation Program: Stage Two
Chef's Menu

Here is our Chef's Menu, from some of the greatest cooks in Paris. Although these recipes (listed by page number) are easy to prepare, they are no less delightful than the finest meals served along the banks of the Seine.

Even if you're not an experienced cook, try some of these recipes. Many are so simple they may turn you into a chef, as well as a successful dieter.

DAY ONE

BREAKFAST
2 slices plain bread (any type)
  with 1 pat butter or
  margarine
½ cup plain low-fat yogurt
½ cup orange juice
beverage

LUNCH
Salade Marignan (Mixed Vegetable
  Salad), page 245
Omelette Soufflée (Fluffy Omelet),
  page 288
1 slice or 1 oz low-fat cheese
  with 1 cracker
½ cup mixed fruit salad
beverage

DINNER
small green salad with 1 tbs light
  dressing
*Poularde en Cocotte aux Senteurs de
  Truffes* (Truffle-Flavored
  Chicken Casserole), page 277
1 slice or 1 oz low-fat cheese
beverage

DAY TWO

BREAKFAST
1 cup any unsweetened cereal
    with ½ cup skim milk, no
    sugar, artificial sweetener
    permitted
½ cup grapefruit juice
beverage

LUNCH
Gâteau de Carottes au Coulis
    d'Asperges (Carrot Cakes with
    Asparagus Sauce), page 258
Fondant de Volaille au Whiskey
    (Chicken Salad with Whiskey
    Dressing), page 282
½ cup plain low-fat yogurt
1 apple
beverage

DINNER
small *salade vermeil* (salad of
    radishes, mushrooms, and
    lemon juice)
Arlequin de Poissons Grillés (Mixed
    Grilled Fish), page 307
2 medium potatoes with 1 pat
    butter or margarine
½ cup plain low-fat yogurt
beverage

DAY THREE

BREAKFAST
2 slices plain bread (any type)
    with 2 pats butter or
    margarine
1 slice or 1 oz low-fat cheese
beverage

LUNCH
small bowl vegetable soup
St. Jacques Lutées (Sealed
    Scallops), page 295
1 cup cooked rice
½ cup low-fat cottage cheese
    with 1 piece chopped fruit
beverage

DINNER
*Méli-Mélo de Crevettes Roses aux
    Huîtres* (Hodgepodge of Pink
    Shrimp with Oysters),
    page 298
Filet de Boeuf Grand-Mère (Old-
    Fashioned Filet of Beef),
    page 265
½ cup plain low-fat yogurt
½ cup oranges (fresh or canned
    in their own juice, not
    sweetened), with fresh mint
beverage

DAY FOUR

BREAKFAST
2 slices plain bread (any type)
    with 1 pat butter or
    margarine
½ cup plain low-fat yogurt
1 orange
beverage

LUNCH
Salade de Haricots Verts Printanière
    (Springtime Green Bean
    Salad), page 246
Escalope de Saumon aux Primeurs
    (Salmon Scallopini with Fresh
    Vegetables), page 291
1 medium boiled potato
1 slice or 1 oz low-fat cheese
beverage

DINNER
small green salad with 1 tbs light
    dressing
*Croquette d'Agneau en Bouquet de
    Légumes* (Lamb with Mixed
    Vegetables), page 270
Yogourt Glacé au Coulis de Kiwi
    (Frozen Yogurt with Kiwi
    Sauce), page 313
beverage

DAY FIVE

BREAKFAST
2 slices plain bread (any type)
   with 1 pat butter or
   margarine
1 slice or 1 oz low-fat cheese
beverage

LUNCH
¼ cup low-fat cottage cheese
   with cucumber slices and
   chives
Filet de Dinde en Habit-Vert
   (Turkey Filet in French
   Academy Costume),
   page 284
½ cup fresh pineapple chunks
beverage

DINNER
Gaspacho de Tomates (Tomato
   Gazpacho), page 243
Émincé de Canard aux Deux Poivres
   (Duck Slivers with Two
   Peppers), page 283
½ cup stewed apples and pears,
   no sugar, artificial sweetener
   permitted
beverage

DAY SIX

BREAKFAST
1 cup any unsweetened cereal
   with ½ cup skim milk, no
   sugar, artificial sweetener
   permitted
½ cup mixed fruit salad
beverage

LUNCH
Soufflé de Brocolis aux Deux Épices
   (Broccoli Soufflé with Two
   Spices), page 256
Parfait de Gambas (Shrimp
   Parfaits), page 297
½ cup purée of celery
2 medium boiled potatoes
½ cup plain low-fat yogurt
beverage

DINNER

small raw mushroom salad with
lemon juice and 1 tbs oil or
regular salad dressing
Sauté de Veau aux Petits Légumes
(Sautéed Veal with
Vegetables), page 268
1 slice or 1 oz low-fat cheese
2 plain crackers
beverage

DAY SEVEN

BREAKFAST
2 slices plain bread (any type)
with 2 pats butter or
margarine
1 egg, any style
1 slice lean ham
beverage

LUNCH
½ pink grapefruit, no sugar,
artificial sweetener permitted
Panaché de Viande Grillée (Mixed
Grilled Meat), page 272
½ cup plain low-fat yogurt
beverage

DINNER

small green salad with 1 tbs oil
or regular salad dressing
*Jambonnette de Volaille au Parfum de
Truffes* (Chicken Flavored with
Truffles), page 275
1 slice or 1 oz low-fat cheese
1 slice plain bread (any type) or
4 plain crackers
Soupe de Fraises au Champagne
(Strawberries in Champagne),
page 312
beverage

DAY EIGHT

BREAKFAST
1 cup any unsweetened cereal
   with ½ cup skim milk, no
   sugar, artificial sweetener
   permitted
½ cup grapefruit juice
beverage

LUNCH
Émincé de Volaille aux Deux Choux
   (Chicken Breasts with
   Broccoli and Cauliflower),
   page 274
½ cup plain low-fat yogurt
beverage

DINNER
small mixed salad with 1 tbs oil
   or regular salad dressing
Filets de Truite aux Petits Légumes
   (Trout Filets with Small
   Vegetables), page 303
1 slice or 1 oz low-fat cheese
1 slice plain bread (any type) or
   4 plain crackers
beverage

DAY NINE

BREAKFAST
2 slices plain bread (any type)
   with 1 pat butter or
   margarine
1 cup plain low-fat yogurt
beverage

LUNCH
small bowl of carrot and
   cucumber sticks, and raw
   cauliflowerets with 1 tbs light
   dressing
Coeur de Filet de Boeuf aux Épices
   (Beef Filet with Spices),
   page 266
Pétales de Kiwi au Jus de Fraises
   (Kiwi Petals with Strawberry
   Purée), page 313
beverage

DINNER

Asperges aux Champignons en Duo
(Duet of Asparagus and
Mushrooms), page 255
*Petite Nage aux Senteurs d'Herbe
Folle* (Mixed Seafood Flavored
with Wild Herbs), page 308
½ cup cooked rice
Orange au Four (Baked Orange),
page 311
½ cup plain low-fat yogurt
beverage

DAY TEN

BREAKFAST

2 slices plain bread (any type)
with 2 pats butter or
margarine
½ cup plain low-fat yogurt
½ cup orange juice
beverage

LUNCH

large green salad with 3 oz
warmed chicken livers and
1 tbs sherry vinegar plus 1 tbs
oil or regular salad dressing
1 slice or 1 oz low-fat cheese
2 slices plain bread (any type) or
8 plain crackers
Pommes Surprises au Four (Baked
Apple Surprise), page 310
beverage

DINNER

small bowl vegetable soup
Rôti de Bar au Varech (Broiled
Bass with Seaweed),
page 289
½ cup plain low-fat yogurt
Brochettes de Fruits en Papillotes
(Fruit Skewers), page 316
beverage

DAY ELEVEN

BREAKFAST
1 cup any unsweetened cereal
  with ½ cup skim milk, no
  sugar, artificial sweetener
  permitted
beverage

LUNCH
small bowl steamed leeks or
  small green salad with
  vinaigrette dressing
*Oeufs Durs ou Pochés Florentine aux
  Épinards* (Hard-Cooked or
  Poached Eggs with Spinach),
  page 287
1 slice or 1 oz low-fat cheese
1 slice plain bread (any type) or
  4 plain crackers
1 pear
beverage

DINNER
medium mixed raw vegetable
  salad with 1 tbs oil or regular
  salad dressing
Poulet Tandoori (Tandoori
  Chicken), page 279
⅔ cup cooked rice
Mousse aux Deux Fruits (Two-Fruit
  Mousse), page 314
beverage

DAY TWELVE

BREAKFAST
2 slices plain bread (any type)
  with 1 pat butter or
  margarine
¾ cup plain low-fat yogurt
1 piece fruit
beverage

LUNCH
small two-toned salad (carrots
  and white cabbage) with 1 tbs
  oil or regular salad dressing
Suprême de Dinde en Papillotes
  (Turkey Supreme in
  Papillotes), page 285
Gratin de Fraises à la Cannelle
  (Cinnamon-Flavored
  Strawberries), page 312
beverage

DINNER

Courgettes aux Crevettes Roses
   (Zucchini with Pink Shrimp),
   page 262
*Médaillons de Langouste aux Vapeurs
   d'Herbes Sauvages* (Medallions
   of Lobster Scented with Wild
   Herbs), page 306
1 medium boiled potato
1 slice or 1 oz low-fat cheese
1 slice plain bread (any type) or
   4 plain crackers
beverage

DAY THIRTEEN

BREAKFAST

2 slices plain bread (any type)
   with 1 pat butter or
   margarine
1 slice or 1 oz low-fat cheese
1 soft-boiled egg
beverage

LUNCH

small green salad with 1 tbs light
   dressing
*Filet de Sole à la Purée de
   Concombre* (Filet of Sole with
   Cucumber Purée), page 301
½ cup low-fat cottage cheese
   with fresh peach slices
beverage

DINNER

4 oz leg of lamb with *Confiture
   d'Oignons Grenadine* (Onion
   Preserve with Grenadine),
   page 254
½ cup steamed green beans
   with parsley
½ cup plain low-fat yogurt
*Aspic de Fruits Frais aux Saveurs
   Exotiques* (Fresh Fruit Aspic
   with Exotic Flavors),
   page 315
beverage

DAY FOURTEEN

BREAKFAST
rice pudding without sugar,
  sweetened with apricots
  canned in their own juice
1 slice or 1 oz low-fat cheese
beverage

LUNCH
small green salad with 1 tbs oil
  or regular salad dressing
Poulet Pané au Sésame (Breaded
  Chicken with Sesame Seeds),
  page 278
½ cup grilled or stewed
  tomatoes
Mousse au Chocolat Noir Allégé
  (Low-Calorie Dark Chocolate
  Mousse), page 316
beverage

DINNER
1 regular slice melon
St. Pierre au Citron Vert et au Coco
  (Grouper with Lime and
  Coconut), page 290
½ cup steamed zucchini and
  eggplant
½ cup cooked rice
½ cup plain low-fat yogurt
beverage

You can follow this menu for only one of the days, on special
occasions, or for the entire two weeks if you want to eat like royalty
while dieting.

PART THREE

--- ❖ ---

The Paris Diet❖
The
Weight Loss
Program

STAGE ONE *(2 weeks)*
STAGE TWO *(2 weeks)*

CHAPTER 7

The Weight Loss Program: Stage One

*H*ere you are, at the most exciting part of the Paris Diet—the Weight Loss Program. Now the extra weight will just melt away. In a few weeks, you'll look better and feel better about yourself. And even though this is the most restricted phase of the diet, you won't be plagued by hunger and feelings of deprivation. If you use the Chef's Recipes, you'll be eating some of the most delicious food you've ever tasted. It's luxurious dining fare designed to make you enjoy losing weight.

First, we want to congratulate you for sticking to the diet. Although you are about to start the hardest part and will restrict your food intake over the next few weeks, we've made it as easy as we can. But it will involve some sacrifices on your part. Look at it this way: The food you'll be eating is good for your health and the way you look. And the end justifies the means: Once you've completed the program, you'll never have to diet again. That should be more than enough incentive to keep you on track.

During the Weight Loss Program, you will be at Stage One, the lowest calorie level (600 calories), for two weeks and then go on to Stage Two with an additional 300 calories for the following two weeks. As we explained earlier, if you are heavy (10 percent or more over your ideal weight) or if you eat over 1,400 calories a day, you should start with this Weight Loss Program of the Paris Diet.

Despite its low-calorie level, the Weight Loss Program won't make you feel uncomfortable. Why? Because at this point the diet is high in protein. This has many advantages:

• you lose fat, not muscle. Some very low-calorie diets result in muscle loss, which leaves you feeling weak and dizzy, and they can even be dangerous;

• protein eliminates the hunger pangs that so often plague dieters and ultimately cause a diet to fail;

• the body uses fewer calories from protein-rich foods than from foods rich in carbohydrate or fat because it becomes less efficient and burns off the extra calories as heat.

All these factors work in your favor when you start this part of the diet. Some other plans use foods that actually make your body work against you and prevent you from losing weight. Or they make you feel so hungry and dizzy you can't take it for more than a few days. Many a diet has ended precisely at this point. This won't happen on the Paris Diet.

Before you start this phase, read the general guidelines in Chapter 4, and follow our advice for using salt, drinking fluids, cooking and preparing food, and so on. Also, remember these things:

1. Take Supplements During This Stage of the Diet

Because you're eating less than normal, your body will need extra vitamins and minerals. The best one-per-day multivitamin supplements are those that come closest to the amounts suggested by the RDA (see the appendix). Don't waste your time and money or endanger your health with megadoses. They're never needed, no matter what the ads say.

You should also take a daily supplement of 500 mg of potassium. Women in particular should take an additional calcium supplement of 1,000 mg daily in the form of calcium carbonate. If you have a vitamin deficiency or take a prescription medication such as a diuretic that could cause vitamin or mineral depletion, make sure you talk to your doctor before starting this stage and ask him which kinds and amounts of supplements you should take. (Besides, as we have mentioned, everyone should consult their physicians before starting any new diet or exercise program.)

2. Eat Three Meals a Day and Avoid Snacking

Make sure you eat three meals per day, preferably at a set time. Don't wait until you're starving to eat (when you're very hungry, invariably you'll eat more than you should). Also, try to avoid snacking. It's a bad habit and can easily add on extra calories. Should you feel hunger cravings, the best way to handle them is to drink a tall glass of water, preferably carbonated.

If you absolutely must have a snack between meals, borrow an item from your daily allowance but remember not to have it twice. For example, if you need a ½ cup of yogurt between meals, eliminate it from the dinner or lunch menu. If you want to snack with your family at night, save your dessert from dinner. Try not to cut food from the breakfast menu—the morning meal is the most important of the day. It provides the fuel you need to get you going and to keep you alert through the working hours.

We can't stress enough how snacking can completely undermine this diet. Now is the best time for you to kick that habit for good.

3. Stick to the Foods and Quantities Indicated—Avoid Those Extras

One reason you shouldn't skip a meal on this plan is that your protein needs will not be taken care of, your hunger will increase, and nibbling might be the result. This stage of the diet is very carefully calculated to maximize weight loss. If you slip and add in extra calories, either by using prohibited foods or by boosting the quantities we've indicated (eating 10 ounces of meat instead of 4), you could raise your caloric intake to the point where you won't lose the weight you want. This diet is as delicate as your own body; stick to the foods and quantities we've indicated as closely as you can, and you'll be thrilled with the results. The Paris Diet is designed to help you avoid temptation by giving you satisfying things to eat—try not to add any more goodies than we've provided.

4. Use Our Sauces and Dressings

On this stage of the diet, you are not allowed to use regular salad dressings. Beware of many low-calorie dressings, as well—they may contain more fat and calories than you think. Check the labels of light dressings, and make sure they don't have more than 25 calories per tablespoon. Use only 1 tablespoon per day. Better still, use our special dressings and sauces (up to 25 calories per day—see calorie counts in the recipes).

During Stage One of the Weight Loss Program, the lightest dressing/sauce you can make is with lemon, herbs, pepper, vinegar, and a small chopped onion (less than 5 calories per tablespoon). Sauces and purées can be made from vegetables. Reduce tomatoes, eggplants, mushrooms, watercress, celery, leeks, and/or diced carrots to a pulp through long, slow cooking, add spices and herbs, then use to season dishes (less than 5 calories per tablespoon). You can also use the following recipes (page numbers are in parentheses):

FOR SALADS
Sauce Verte/Green Dressing (page 252)
Sauce Menthe/Mint Vinegar (page 248)
Sauce Sontay/Creamy Spinach Dressing (page 249)
Sauce Yogourt/Yogurt Sauce (page 249)
Sauce Tomates aux Aromates/Spicy Tomato Sauce (page 253)
Vinaigre Zéro/Red Vinaigrette (page 247)

FOR VEGETABLES AND FISH
Sauce Maraîchère/Tomato and Lemon Sauce with Herbs (page 253)

FOR ZUCCHINI, COLD MEAT, AND FISH
Sauce Tomates à la Chinoise/Chinese-Style Tomato Sauce (page 254)

5. *On This Stage of the Program, Avoid Strenuous Exercise*
During the Weight Loss Program, you are taking in fewer calories than normal. Thus, you should eliminate all strenuous forms of exercise. Do easy stretches and workouts, such as a half hour of walking each day. For more on exercise, see Chapter 12.

6. *You're Not Losing Food*
The foods allowed during the Weight Loss Program are basically the same as those at the higher calorie levels. You're really not depriving yourself of flavors! The only differences are in the starch

and fat categories; the higher calorie levels add breads, rice, pasta, potatoes, starchy vegetables, and some oil, butter, margarine, and cream.

The following tables list the authorized and prohibited foods.

The Weight Loss Program

Prohibited Foods

For easier selection, here is a list of foods you cannot eat during the Weight Loss Program. Although it may seem as if you have lost a lot, you can still have great meals. Our special dressings and sauces make most foods taste delicious and satisfying. If you try some of our recipes, you can be eating dishes and desserts like Chicken Flavored with Truffles, Scallops Gratin with a Fringe of Endives, Sole with Grapes, Kiwi Petals in Strawberry Purée, and Dark Chocolate Mousse.

A prohibited food will occasionally be included, however, to give your mind and taste buds a treat, but don't add one yourself. Follow the meal plans carefully, and only add indulgences where we've indicated.

SUGAR AND SWEETENED PRODUCTS
sugar, honey, jams, "diet jams," jellies, cookies, pastries, ice cream, sherbet, candies, chocolate, chocolate-flavored drinks, chewing gum with sugar, sorbitol or xylitol (sweeteners that contain significant calories), yogurt or other dairy products with flavorings or fruit added, candied fruit, fruit in syrup, canned fruit compote, dried fruits (apricots, dates, figs, prunes, raisins, etc.), syrups, canned or bottled fruit juices, soda, cereal bars

STARCHES
breads, flaky rolls, crackers, melba toast, breadsticks, matzo, cocktail snack crackers, cereals, pasta, rice, semolina, potatoes, dried legumes (white beans, lentils, split peas, chick peas)

ALCOHOL
all, including flambéed meats, wine sauces, etc.

FATTY FOODS

sauces, fried foods, French fries, potato chips, doughnuts, pizza, quiche, avocados, and anything cooked with oil or fat

Deli Meats: pâté, salami, bologna, frankfurters, sausages, wursts, corned beef, pastrami, tongue

Fatty Meats: pork, mutton, lamb, duck, goose, venison, fatty cuts of beef (like filet mignon or chuck)

Fish and Shellfish: eel, lamprey, breaded fish, fish canned in oil, clams, oysters

Dairy Foods with high fat content: Cheeses with greater than 50 percent fat content: Roquefort, Gorgonzola, bleu, Brillat-Savarin, St. Andre, Boursault, Caprice des Dieux, regular and goat cheeses with boosted cream content, creamed cheese, creamed Swiss cheese; regular or creamed cottage cheese or yogurt, whole milk

Nuts: almonds, peanuts, hazelnuts, walnuts, cashews, pine nuts, Brazils, etc.

Authorized Foods

Here are the foods you can eat. If you think the prohibited list cut out all delightful foods, think again. There's plenty left, and all of it healthy for mind, body, and figure. Try our special sauces and dressings to add bulk and flavoring to any meal. Steamed Baby Lobster with Vegetables, and Fresh Fruit Aspic with Exotic Flavors are just two of the dishes you and your family can enjoy—even on this stage of the program.

LEAN, TRIMMED MEATS

beef, veal, chicken (all poultry to be eaten without skin), pheasant, turkey and chicken cutlets, roast turkey, rabbit, lean lamb; very lean roast pork, filet of pork or pork chops can be eaten once a week

LEAN FISH

cod, haddock, pollack, lemon sole, sole, bass, whiting, ray, red mullet, red snapper, turbot

FATTY FISH

shad, anchovies, carp, herring, lake trout, mackerel, sardines, salmon, tuna, all packed in water (no oil)

> EAT FISH, LEAN OR FATTY, SEVERAL TIMES EACH WEEK

FRESH FRUITS AND VEGETABLES

DAIRY FOODS, LOW FAT

Cheeses with less than 50 percent fat content: low-fat Camembert, Comte, Coulommiers, low-fat Brie, Gruyère, Port du Salut, Edam, Gouda, Mimolette, Cheshire, low-fat goat cheese, Roblochon, Saint-Nectaire, Tomme; 1-2 percent low-fat plain yogurt, low-fat plain cottage cheese

You're now ready to start Stage One of the Weight Loss Program. The Paris Diet offers you three menu choices. You can follow the Summary Plan, which tells you the basic foods and amounts you have to eat. Use the following exchange (equivalency) tables. They list foods that are the exact equals, calorie-wise, of others.

You might follow the Standard Diet, which gives you two weeks of simple, yet appetizing meals. If you love fine food, try our Chef's Menu, which comes from some of the finest professional cooks in Paris!

You also could combine them. For example, you might follow the Summary Plan for busy days or at a restaurant; the Standard Diet for evening meals or lazy days around the house; and the Chef's Menu for weekends or whenever you want gourmet meals that are quick and easy to prepare.

The Weight Loss Program: Exchange (Equivalency) Tables

The following tables list foods in different categories that are approximately the same, calorie-wise, as other foods. You should use them in two ways. First, these tables will form the basis of the Summary Plan. If lunch calls for ½ cup of cooked vegetables, just look at the vegetable exchange list to see which ones you can choose from.

You can also use these lists to vary your diet if you are following the set menu plans. This is advisable since boredom sabotages any regimen. Simply pick a food from the lists that equals the one in the plan and substitute it. Make sure you use the quantity listed or it won't be equal in caloric value to the food for which it's being exchanged. For example, if you don't feel like having ½ cup of beets, exchange it for 6 ounces of tomato juice—not 4 or 8 ounces but 6 ounces.

Not all foods in the menu plans will have exchanges.

Each one of the foods contained within a numbered list is equal to all others in that list. You can also choose to make two exchanges: For instance, if you want to eat 1 apple, you can either exchange it for 1 small banana, or for 10 cherries plus ½ cup of orange juice. It's up to you.

If the menu calls for 4 ounces of beef, and the exchange table lists beef in quantities of 1 ounce, remember to multiply all the other quantities in the list by 4 if you are exchanging for the beef. In other words, since 1 ounce of beef equals 1 slice of low-fat cheese, 4 ounces of beef would be equal to 4 slices of low-fat cheese.

I. Vegetable Exchanges (for ½ cup cooked or 1 cup raw)

asparagus
beans (green or wax)
bean sprouts
beets
broccoli
Brussels sprouts
cabbage (all kinds)
carrots
catsup, 2 tablespoons
cauliflower
celery
cucumber

eggplant
leafy greens (all kinds)
mushrooms
okra
onion
pepper (red or green)
rutabaga
sauerkraut
squash, summer
tomato
tomato or vegetable juice,
   6 ounces

II. Fruit Exchanges

FRUITS
apple, ½ medium
applesauce, ½ cup

apricots, dried, 4 halves
apricots, fresh, 2 medium

banana, ½ small

blueberries, ½ cup

cantaloupe (6-inch diameter),
   ¼ medium

cherries, 10 large

dates, 2

figs, dried, 1 small

fruit cocktail, canned, ½ cup

grapefruit, ½ small

grapes, 15 small

honeydew melon (7-inch
   diameter), ⅓

mango, ½ small

nectarine, 1 small

orange, 1 small

papaya, ⅓ medium

peach, 1 medium

pear, 1 small

pineapple, ½ cup

prunes, dried, 2

raisins, 2 tablespoons

strawberries, ¾ cup

tangerine, 1 large

watermelon, 1 cup cubed

JUICES

apple, pineapple,
grapefruit, orange, ½ cup

grape, prune, ¼ cup

III. Starch Exchanges (cooked servings)

BREADS

bagel, ½

bun for hamburger or
   hot dog, ½

cornbread (1½-inch diameter),
   1 cube

dinner roll (2-inch diameter), 1

English muffin, ½

plain bread (no honey or fruit
   added), 1 slice

tortilla (6-inch diameter), 1

CRACKERS

graham (2½-inch square), 2

matzo (4 by 6 inches), ½

melba toast, 4

oyster crackers (½ cup), 20

pretzels, 8 rings

rye krisps, 3

saltines, 5

CEREALS

bran, 5 tablespoons

dry flakes, ⅔ cup

dry puffed, 1½ cups

hot cereal such as oatmeal,
   farina, ½ cup

pastas, ½ cup

rice, ½ cup

wheat germ, 2 tablespoons

STARCHY VEGETABLES

beans or peas (plain),
   ½ cup

corn, ⅓ cup or ½ medium ear

parsnips, ⅔ cup

potatoes, white, 1 small or   pumpkin, ¾ cup
   ½ cup   squash, winter, ½ cup
potatoes, sweet or yams, ¼ cup
DESSERTS
angel cake, 1½ inch square   fat-free sherbet, 4 ounces

IV. Protein Exchanges (cooked weight)
beef, dried, chipped, 1 ounce   fish, 1 ounce
beef, lamb, pork, veal (lean   lobster, 1 small tail
   only), 1 ounce   oysters, clams, shrimps,
cheese, hard, ½ ounce   5 medium
cheese, low fat, 1 ounce or   peanut butter, 2 teaspoons
   1 slice   poultry, without skin, 1 ounce
cottage cheese, plain, low fat,   salmon, pink, canned, ¼ cup
   ¼ cup*   tuna, packed in water, ¼ cup
egg, 1 medium

V. Dairy Exchanges
cheese, hard, ½ ounce   milk, 1% fat, ½ cup
cheese, low fat, 1 ounce or   milk, skim, ⅔ cup
   1 slice   yogurt, plain, low fat, ½ cup
cottage cheese, plain, low fat,
   ¼ cup

VI. Fat Exchanges
avocado (4-inch diameter), ⅛   olives, 5 small
bacon, crisp, 1 slice   peanuts, 10
butter or margarine, 1 pat   Roquefort dressing, 1 tablespoon
French dressing, 1 tablespoon   Thousand Island dressing,
mayonnaise, 2 teaspoons   1 tablespoon
oil, 2 teaspoons (all kinds)   walnuts, 6 small

   * Note: Cheeses contain good amounts of protein and calcium; therefore,
they are listed in two tables and can be used either as an exchange for a protein-
rich food or as an exchange for a dairy food.

The Weight Loss Program: Stage One
Summary for Easy Reference

On this stage of the diet, you will eat certain basic foods each day. If you don't want to follow the Standard Diet or Chef's Menu, use this summary for any or all of the days. You might choose to follow the Chef's Menu on the weekends, but on a busy Monday, substitute the simple foods listed below.

Refer to the exchange tables to find out which foods are the exact equivalents of the ones below. If you do make a substitution, use the exact quantities in the tables. For example, 1 cup of plain low-fat yogurt is equal to 1⅓ cups of skim milk. You could eat either and adhere to the diet. However, if you drink 2 cups of skim milk in place of 1 cup of yogurt, you'd be consuming too many calories.

You might want to photocopy the summary page to have it with you when you're away from home, so you'll never be in doubt about how much and what to eat.

The Weight Loss Program: Stage One

Summary Plan

BREAKFAST

½ cup plain low-fat yogurt or ½ cup low-fat cottage cheese
½ cup unsweetened fruit juice or 1 piece of fruit (can be saved for
   dessert at lunch or dinner)
beverage

LUNCH

small green salad with 1 tbs light dressing
½ cup cooked vegetable (boiled or steamed without oil or fat) or
   1 cup raw vegetables
4 oz lean meat or fish (cooked without oil or fat—baked,
   broiled, steamed, or grilled only)
beverage

DINNER

small green salad with 1 tbs light dressing
½ cup cooked vegetables (boiled or steamed without oil or fat) or
   1 cup raw vegetables
4 oz lean meat or fish (cooked without oil or fat—baked, broiled,
   steamed, or grilled only)
½ cup plain low-fat yogurt or ½ cup low-fat cottage cheese
beverage

For Men

Since men have more muscle mass and therefore slightly higher
protein needs than women, men must add one of the following:

2 whites of eggs (no yolks), hard-boiled, chopped into salads, or
¼ cup low-fat cottage cheese, or
½ cup plain low-fat yogurt

These extra foods can be eaten at any point in the day and should
be added to the Summary Plan, Standard Diet, and Chef's Menu.

The Weight Loss Program: Stage One
Cold Meals You Can Take to Work

With our busy schedules, many of us don't have time to prepare elaborate lunches or go out to restaurants. Therefore, the following are some examples of cold meals for lunch or early dinner that you may easily prepare at home and take to the office. By following the Summary Plan, you may also come up with your own ideas for simple bagable items—just make sure you stick to the basic guidelines.

MEAL #1
small raw vegetable salad with
  1 tbs light dressing
1 roast chicken leg or 4 oz white
  meat chicken
1 apple (you'll skip it at
  breakfast)
beverage

MEAL #2
2 stalks celery chopped with
  1 tbs light dressing
2 slices cold lean meat
½ cup plain low-fat yogurt or
  ½ cup low-fat cottage cheese
  (you'll skip it at dinner)
beverage

MEAL #3
small bowl cucumber salad with
  1 tbs light dressing
4 oz lean white fish
½ cup plain low-fat yogurt or
  ½ cup low-fat cottage cheese
  (you'll skip it at dinner)
beverage

MEAL #4
small to medium mixed salad
  (diced hard low-fat cheese,
  small dices of ham, plain tuna
  fish, spices, baby onions) with
  1 tbs light dressing
1 apple or 1 pear or 3 small
  apricots (you'll skip it at
  breakfast)
beverage

(You might also want to pack any cold meals from the Standard Diet or even the Chef's Menu, and any hot meals if there's a microwave at work.)

The Weight Loss Program: Stage One

The Standard Diet

The following menu plans are for two weeks of the 600-calorie Standard Diet, which you will find tasty and satisfying. All foods are simple to find and prepare. However, if you want to add a little gourmet flavor, we have included some quick and easy recipes you can substitute in place of the regular meals. These recipes can be found on the pages listed in the menu plans.

Whether you stick to the basic foods or include a recipe or two, you'll now start to lose the weight you want. And best of all, you won't regain it after a few months!

DAY ONE

BREAKFAST
½ cup plain low-fat yogurt
½ cup unsweetened grapefruit
    juice
beverage

LUNCH
2 eggs, any style, with ½ cup
    cooked peppers (or *Oeufs Durs
    ou Pochés Florentine aux
    Épinards*/Hard-Cooked or
    Poached Eggs with Spinach,
    page 287)
½ cup low-fat cottage cheese
beverage

DINNER
medium green salad with 1 tbs
    light dressing
4 oz lean steak
½ cup stewed tomatoes, cooked
    carrots, or cooked spinach (or
    ½ cup *Tomates Provençale/*
    Provence-Style Tomatoes,
    page 259)
beverage

DAY TWO

BREAKFAST
½ cup low-fat cottage cheese
beverage

LUNCH
small mixed salad with tomato,
　　lettuce, and cucumber and
　　1 tbs light dressing (or
　　Carottes Vichy/Sliced Carrots
　　with Parsley, page 257)
4 oz lean hamburger
½ cup plain low-fat yogurt
beverage

DINNER
4 oz flounder or other white fish
　　with ½ cup cooked mixed
　　vegetables, green beans, or
　　spinach (or *Pot-au-Feu de la
　　Mer*/Fish Stew with Herbs,
　　page 309)
1 orange
beverage

DAY THREE

BREAKFAST
1 oz low-fat cheese with 1 rice
　　cake
½ cup orange juice
beverage

LUNCH
4 oz broiled or cold skinless
　　chicken breast with ½ cup
　　cooked tomatoes (or *Poulet
　　Basquaise*/Stewed Chicken
　　Basque Style, page 280)
beverage

DINNER
4 oz grilled veal chop
½ cup cooked green beans or
　　Brussels sprouts or 6 spears
　　steamed asparagus
½ cup low-fat cottage cheese
beverage

DAY FOUR

BREAKFAST
½ cup plain low-fat yogurt
beverage

LUNCH
4 oz lean cold cuts: any
    combination of turkey, roast
    beef, or ham with small
    mixed salad and dressing (or
    Courgettes Farcies/Stuffed
    Zucchini, page 260)
1 oz low-fat cheese
beverage

DINNER
small mixed salad of tomatoes
    and cucumber with 1 tbs
    light dressing
4 oz sole or other white fish
1 apple
beverage

DAY FIVE

BREAKFAST
1 egg, any style
½ cup orange juice
beverage

LUNCH
small chef's salad (1 slice of
    chicken, turkey, lean ham,
    tomato, salad greens) with
    1 tbs light dressing
½ cup plain low-fat yogurt
beverage

DINNER
4 oz lean pork
1¼ cups steamed broccoli,
    cauliflower, or cabbage
1 oz low-fat cheese with 1 rice
    cake
beverage

DAY SIX

BREAKFAST
½ cup plain low-fat yogurt
beverage

LUNCH
3–4 oz individual can of water-
 packed tuna
1 medium tomato, ½ cup raw
 celery, or ½ small cucumber
 with 1 tbs light dressing
½ cup sherbet flavored with
 artificial sweetener
beverage

DINNER
4 oz lamb cutlets with ½ cup
 cooked squash or broccoli (or
 *Sauté de Veau aux Petits
 Légumes*/Sautéed Veal with
 Vegetables, page 268)
½ cup low-fat cottage cheese
beverage

DAY SEVEN

BREAKFAST
½ cup plain low-fat yogurt
½ cup grapefruit juice
beverage

LUNCH
large mixed salad with 1 tbs
 light dressing
4 oz cold meat with 1 tbs light
 sauce
beverage

DINNER
½ cup low-fat cottage cheese
 with chives and cucumber
 slices
4 oz broiled skinless turkey
½ cup cooked green beans,
 boiled spinach or cooked
 zucchini
beverage

DAY EIGHT

BREAKFAST
½ cup low-fat cottage cheese
apricots, 2 medium fresh or 4
    halves canned in own juice
beverage

LUNCH
medium green salad with 1 tbs
    light dressing
4 oz grilled or broiled
    hamburger
½ cup plain low-fat yogurt
beverage

DINNER
small green salad with 1 tbs light
    dressing
4 oz broiled veal chop
½ cup cooked green beans,
    Brussels sprouts, or broccoli
beverage

DAY NINE

BREAKFAST
½ cup plain low-fat yogurt
beverage

LUNCH
2 eggs, any style, with 1 baked
    tomato (or *Piperade*/Scrambled
    Eggs with Tomatoes and
    Sweet Peppers, page 286)
½ cup pineapple-flavored low-
    fat cottage cheese
beverage

DINNER
4 oz filet of sole or other white
    fish
½ cup cooked spinach, peas, or
    carrots
beverage

DAY TEN

BREAKFAST
½ cup low-fat cottage cheese
½ cup orange juice
beverage

LUNCH
medium chef's salad (1 slice of
    chicken, turkey, lean ham,
    tomato, salad greens) with
    1 tbs light dressing
beverage

DINNER
medium green salad with 1 tbs
    light dressing
4 oz broiled lean steak
½ cup plain low-fat yogurt
beverage

DAY ELEVEN

BREAKFAST
½ cup plain low-fat yogurt with
    1 piece chopped fresh fruit
beverage

LUNCH
4 oz lean hamburger
½ cup cooked green peas or
    carrots
¼ cup low-fat cottage cheese
beverage

DINNER
medium green salad with 1 tbs
    light dressing
4 oz chicken breast with ½ cup
    steamed mixed vegetables
beverage

DAY TWELVE

BREAKFAST
1 slice low-fat cheese
½ cup grapefruit juice
beverage

LUNCH
3–4 oz individual can of water-
    packed tuna or salmon, with
    small mixed salad and
    dressing (or *Moules Marinières/*
    Steamed Mussels, page 293)
½ cup plain low-fat yogurt
beverage

DINNER
1 cup clear broth (not chunky or
    creamy soup)
medium green salad with 1 tbs
    light dressing
4 oz broiled lean steak with
    ½ cup cooked mushrooms,
    tomatoes, or peppers
beverage

DAY THIRTEEN

BREAKFAST
½ cup low-fat cottage cheese
beverage

LUNCH
large green salad with 1 tbs light
    dressing
4 oz cold skinless chicken (or
    *Émincé de Veau à la Sauge/*Veal
    Cutlets with Sage, page 269)
½ cup plain low-fat yogurt
beverage

DINNER
small mixed salad with dressing
    (or *Salade Maraîchère/*Raw
    Vegetable Salad, page 244)
4 oz broiled sole or flounder
6 steamed asparagus tips or

½ cup cooked squash or
mixed vegetables
1 orange
beverage

DAY FOURTEEN

BREAKFAST
½ cup plain low-fat yogurt
½ cup orange juice
beverage

LUNCH
4 oz turkey breast
½ cup cooked broccoli or
spinach
½ large cantaloupe
beverage

DINNER
medium green salad with 1 tbs
light dressing
4 oz lean ham
½ cup cooked tomatoes or corn
(or *Ratatouille*/Stewed
Vegetables Mediterranean
Style, page 263)
½ cup low-fat cottage cheese
beverage

The Weight Loss Program: Stage One
Chef's Menu

Ever think you'd eat gourmet food on a very low calorie diet? Read on! Below is the jewel of the Paris Diet—our Chef's Menu. From some of the most celebrated masters of Parisian kitchens comes an alternate plan for food lovers who also need to lose weight.

By the way, even if you find it easier to follow the Summary Plan or Standard Diet, try to incorporate a few of the chef's recipes into the week. The more delicious the diet, the easier it will be to follow. These recipes can be found on the pages listed in the menu plans.

DAY ONE

BREAKFAST
½ cup plain low-fat yogurt or
    low-fat cottage cheese
beverage

LUNCH
Omelette Soufflée (Fluffy Omelet),
    page 288
½ cup low-fat cottage cheese
beverage

DINNER
small green salad with 1 tbs light
    dressing
*Filet de Sole à la Purée de
    Concombre* (Filet of Sole with
    Cucumber Purée), page 301
*Aspic de Fruits Frais aux Saveurs
    Exotiques* (Fresh Fruit Aspic
    with Exotic Flavors),
    page 315
beverage

DAY TWO

BREAKFAST
½ cup plain low-fat yogurt or
    low-fat cottage cheese
beverage

LUNCH
Asperges aux Champignons en Duo
    (Duet of Asparagus and
    Mushrooms), page 255
*Jambonnette de Volaille au Parfum de
    Truffes* (Chicken Flavored with
    Truffles), page 275
½ cup purée of green beans
beverage

DINNER
small green salad with 1 tbs light
    dressing
Courgettes Farcies (Stuffed
    Zucchini), page 260

> *Yogourt Glacé au Coulis de Kiwi*
> (Frozen Yogurt with Kiwi
> Sauce), page 313
> beverage

DAY THREE

BREAKFAST
½ cup plain low-fat yogurt or
   low-fat cottage cheese
beverage

LUNCH
Salade Marignan (Mixed Vegetable
   Salad), page 245
1 slice lean ham
beverage

DINNER
½ cup low-fat cottage cheese
   with herbs and cucumber
   slices
shish kebab of 4 oz fish (red
   snapper, sole, etc.), tomatoes,
   peppers on a skewer
Pommes Surprises au Four (Baked
   Apple Surprise), page 310
beverage

DAY FOUR

BREAKFAST
½ cup plain low-fat yogurt or
   low-fat cottage cheese
beverage

LUNCH
medium chef's salad (greens,
   tomatoes, cold chicken, hard-
   boiled egg) with 1 tbs light
   dressing
1 pear
beverage

DINNER
Soufflé de Brocolis aux Deux Épices
   (Broccoli Soufflé with Two
   Spices), page 256

DINNER (*cont'd*)
2 thin slices of turkey
½ cup plain low-fat yogurt
beverage

DAY FIVE

BREAKFAST
½ cup plain low-fat yogurt or
   low-fat cottage cheese
½ cup grapefruit juice
beverage

LUNCH
Gaspacho de Tomates (Tomato
   Gazpacho), page 243
*Oeufs Durs ou Pochés Florentine aux
   Épinards* (Hard-Cooked or
   Poached Eggs with Spinach),
   page 287
beverage

DINNER
small green salad with 1 tbs light
   dressing
mixed grill (assorted shish
   kebabs—4 oz fish, turkey,
   chicken, or beef and tomatoes
   and peppers on a skewer)
beverage

DAY SIX

BREAKFAST
½ cup plain low-fat yogurt or
   low-fat cottage cheese
beverage

LUNCH
small green salad with 1 tbs light
   dressing
*Gratin de St. Jacques à l'Effiloché
   d'Endives* (Scallops Gratin with
   a Fringe of Endive), page 294
Soupe de Fraises au Champagne
   (Strawberries in Champagne),
   page 312
beverage

DINNER

small watercress salad with 1 tbs
 light dressing
4 oz grilled veal chop
½ cup low-fat cottage cheese
beverage

DAY SEVEN

BREAKFAST

½ cup plain low-fat yogurt or
 low-fat cottage cheese
beverage

LUNCH

4 oz grilled lean steak
½ cup cooked green peas
½ cup plain low-fat yogurt
beverage

DINNER

Truite au Sel (Trout in Salt),
 page 304
½ cup cooked mixed vegetables
Mousse au Chocolat Noir Allégé
 (Low-Calorie Dark Chocolate
 Mousse), page 316
beverage

DAY EIGHT

BREAKFAST

½ cup plain low-fat yogurt or
 low-fat cottage cheese
beverage

LUNCH

½ cup steamed leeks with
 lemon juice
2 hard-boiled eggs with 1 tbs
 light sauce or dressing
1 slice low-fat cheese
beverage

DINNER

Courgettes aux Crevettes Roses
 (Zucchini with Pink Shrimp),
 page 262
4 oz roast chicken

DINNER (cont'd)
Brochettes de Fruits en Papillottes
   (Fruit Skewers), page 316
beverage

DAY NINE

BREAKFAST
½ cup plain low-fat yogurt or
   low-fat cottage cheese
beverage

LUNCH
small mixed salad (tomato,
   greens, cucumber) with 1 tbs
   light dressing
Sole aux Raisins (Sole with
   Grapes), page 302
beverage

DINNER
small green bean salad with
   1 tbs light dressing
4 oz cold roast beef
½ cup plain low-fat yogurt
beverage

DAY TEN

BREAKFAST
½ cup plain low-fat yogurt or
   low-fat cottage cheese
1 soft-boiled egg
beverage

LUNCH
½ cup raw mushrooms with
   lemon juice
Fondant de Volaille au Whisky
   (Chicken Salad with Whiskey
   Dressing), page 282
½ cup plain low-fat yogurt
beverage

DINNER
Petit Homard à la Vapeur (Steamed
   Baby Lobster with
   Vegetables), page 305
Pétales de Kiwi au Jus de Fraises
   (Kiwi Petals with Strawberry
   Purée), page 313
beverage

DAY ELEVEN

BREAKFAST
½ cup plain low-fat yogurt or
  low-fat cottage cheese
½ cup grapefruit juice
beverage

LUNCH
4 oz red snapper baked in foil
½ cup mixed vegetables
½ cup low-fat cottage cheese
beverage

DINNER
*Pilon de Volaille Cuit au Senteur
  d'Estragon* (Tarragon-Flavored
  Chicken), page 276
½ cup cauliflower purée
beverage

DAY TWELVE

BREAKFAST
½ cup plain low-fat yogurt or
  low-fat cottage cheese
beverage

LUNCH
small green salad with 1 tbs light
  dressing
4 oz total assortment of cold
  meats (1 oz ham, 1 oz roast
  beef, 1 oz roast pork, 1 oz
  turkey)
Mousse aux Deux Fruits (Two-Fruit
  Mousse), page 314
beverage

DINNER
4 oz poached haddock or sole
½ cup steamed spinach or
  1 cup raw spinach with
  1 tbs light dressing
½ cup plain low-fat yogurt
beverage

DAY THIRTEEN

BREAKFAST
½ cup plain low-fat yogurt or
    low-fat cottage cheese
beverage

LUNCH
Cocktail de Crevettes au Soja
    (Shrimp Salad with Sprouts),
    page 299
½ cup plain low-fat yogurt
beverage

DINNER
Filet de Boeuf Grand-Mère (Old-
    Fashioned Filet of Beef),
    page 265
*Aspic de Fruits Frais aux Saveurs
    Exotiques* (Fresh Fruit Aspic
    with Exotic Flavors),
    page 315
beverage

DAY FOURTEEN

BREAKFAST
½ cup plain low-fat yogurt or
    low-fat cottage cheese
beverage

LUNCH
Poulet Pané au Sésame (Breaded
    Chicken with Sesame Seeds),
    page 278
½ cup steamed cauliflower
¾ cup fresh strawberries
beverage

DINNER
4 large grilled shrimp
1 cup steamed mixed vegetables
½ cup plain low-fat yogurt
beverage

CHAPTER 8

The Weight Loss Program:
Stage Two

*C*ongratulations! You have completed Stage One of the Weight Loss Program and by now have lost weight. You are now ready to increase your food intake by 300 calories. You will continue to lose weight even though you're eating more because the Paris Diet uses specific foods and menus that gently enable your body to adjust to a greater amount of food. Stay on this plan for two weeks.

During Stage Two, use the suggestions in Chapter 4 and for Stage One of the Weight Loss Program. Refer to the lists of prohibited and authorized foods, as well as to the exchange tables, in the previous chapter.

On this stage, remember:

1. Don't add salt.
2. Drink plenty of fluids (water, coffee, tea).
3. Don't drink alcohol.
4. In three well-spaced meals, eat all the foods listed for each day, in the amounts listed.
5. Try to avoid snacking; if you must snack, take a treat from the lunch or dinner menu, then cut it from lunch or dinner.
6. Avoid strenuous physical exercise; use our light workouts or ½ hour of normal walking (see Chapter 12).
7. Cook without oil or fat.
8. Don't use sugar; artificial sweeteners are permitted.
9. Continue to take:

• Your daily vitamin and mineral supplement (containing approximately the values for nutrients in the RDA—see appendix, page 318).

• 500 mg of potassium daily;
• 1,000 mg of calcium daily in the form of calcium carbonate (especially important for women).

10. As often as possible, use the chef's recipes—the diet will be more appetizing and therefore easier to follow.

11. Use our light dressings and sauces to add bulk and flavor to salads and meals, but don't use more than 25 calories per day (check recipes and labels of light dressings for the calorie content). Now you can use the following dressings and sauces:

The lightest dressing/sauce you can make is with lemon, herbs, pepper, vinegar, and a small chopped onion (less than 5 calories per tablespoon). Sauces and purées can be made from vegetables. Reduce tomatoes, eggplants, mushrooms, watercress, celery, leeks, and/or diced carrots to a pulp through long, slow cooking, add spices and herbs, then use to season dishes (less than 5 calories per tablespoon). You can also use the following recipes (page numbers are in parentheses).

FOR SALADS
Sauce Verte/Green Dressing (page 252)
Sauce Menthe/Mint Vinegar (page 248)
Sauce Sontay/Creamy Spinach Dressing (page 249)
Sauce Yogourt/Yogurt Sauce (page 249)
Sauce Tomates aux Aromates/Spicy Tomato Sauce (page 253)
Vinaigre Zéro/Red Vinaigrette (page 247)
Sauce Roquefort/Roquefort Cheese Dressing (page 252)
Sauce Grande Bêche/Watercress Dressing (page 250)

FOR SALADS, POULTRY, VEAL, AND BOILED FISH
Sauce Aïoli/Creamed Garlic Dressing (page 250)

FOR VEGETABLES AND FISH
Sauce Maraîchère/Tomato and Lemon Sauce with Herbs (page 253)

FOR ZUCCHINI, COLD MEAT, AND FISH
Sauce Tomates à la Chinoise/Chinese-Style Tomato Sauce (page 254)

The Weight Loss Program: Stage Two

Summary for Easy Reference

On this stage of the diet, you will eat certain basic foods each day. If you don't want to follow the Standard Diet or Chef's Menu, use this summary for any or all of the days. You might choose to follow the Chef's Menu on the weekends, but on a busy Monday, substitute the simple foods listed below.

Refer to the exchange tables on pages 125–28 to find out which foods are the exact equivalents of the ones below. If you do make a substitution, use the exact quantities in the tables. For example, 1 cup of plain low-fat yogurt is equal to 1⅓ cups of skim milk. You could eat either and adhere to the diet. However, if you drink 2 cups of skim milk in place of 1 cup of yogurt, you'd be consuming too many calories.

You might want to photocopy the summary page to have it with you when you're away from home, so you'll never be in doubt about how much and what to eat.

The Weight Loss Program: Stage Two

Summary Plan

BREAKFAST

½ cup plain low-fat yogurt or low-fat cottage cheese
½ cup unsweetened fruit juice or 1 piece of fruit (can be saved for
    dessert at lunch or dinner)
beverage

LUNCH

medium green salad with 1 tbs light dressing
½ cup cooked vegetables (boiled or steamed without oil or fat) or
    1 cup raw vegetables
4 oz lean meat or fish (cooked without oil or fat, baked, broiled,
    steamed, or grilled only)
1 oz low-fat cheese
beverage

DINNER

medium green salad with 1 tbs light dressing
¾ cup cooked vegetables (boiled or steamed without oil or fat) or
    1½ cups raw vegetables
4 oz lean meat or fish (cooked without oil or fat, baked, broiled,
    steamed, or grilled only)
½ cup plain low-fat yogurt or low-fat cottage cheese
1 medium fruit
beverage

For Men

Since men have more muscle mass and therefore slightly higher
protein needs than women, men must add one of the following:

2 whites of eggs (no yolks), hard-boiled, chopped into salads, or
¼ cup low-fat cottage cheese, or
½ cup plain low-fat yogurt

These extra foods can be eaten at any point in the day and should
be added to the Summary Plan, Standard Diet, and Chef's Menu.

The Weight Loss Program: Stage Two

Cold Meals You Can Take to Work

With our busy schedules, many of us don't have time to prepare elaborate lunches or go out to restaurants. Therefore, the following are some examples of cold meals for lunch or early dinner that you may easily prepare at home and take to the office. By following the Summary Plan, you may also come up with your own ideas for simple bagable items—just make sure you stick to the basic guidelines.

MEAL #1
small bowl cucumber salad with
  1 tbs light dressing
1 roast chicken leg or 4 oz white
  meat chicken
1 oz low-fat cheese
1 pear or orange
beverage

MEAL #2
mixed salad (1 oz diced low-fat
  cheese, small dices of ham
  and several flakes of plain,
  water-packed tuna fish) with
  1 tbs light dressing
½ cup plain low-fat yogurt
1 fruit
beverage

MEAL #3
raw mixed vegetable salad with
  1 tbs light dressing
2 thin slices ham or two hard-
  boiled eggs
1 oz low-fat cheese
1 fruit
beverage

(You might also want to pack any cold meals from the Standard Diet or even the Chef's Menu, and any hot meals if there's a microwave at work.)

The Weight Loss Program: Stage Two

The Standard Diet

The following menu plans are for two weeks of the 900-calorie
Standard Diet. Once again, all the foods are simple to find and
prepare, but if you want to add that gourmet touch without too
much extra work, use our recipe suggestions (in parentheses) in place
of the regular meals. These recipes can be found on the pages listed
in the menu plans.

Remember to follow this plan for fourteen days. You've come this
far—you can do it! Large, luscious meals are right around the corner.

DAY ONE

BREAKFAST
½ cup plain low-fat yogurt
½ cup unsweetened grapefruit
    juice
beverage

LUNCH
2 eggs, any style, with ½ cup
    cooked peppers (or *Oeufs Durs*
    ou Pochés Florentine aux
    Épinards/Hard-Cooked or
    Poached Eggs with Spinach,
    page 287)
½ cup low-fat cottage cheese
    with 1 piece chopped fruit
beverage

DINNER
medium green salad with 1 tbs
    light dressing
4 oz lean steak
¾ cup stewed tomatoes, cooked
    carrots, or cooked spinach (or
    ¾ cup *Tomates Provençale*/
    Provence-Style Tomatoes,
    page 259)
1 oz low-fat cheese
beverage

DAY TWO

BREAKFAST
½ cup low-fat cottage cheese
½ cup unsweetened grapefruit
  juice
beverage

LUNCH
4 oz lean hamburger with 1 slice
  of low-fat cheese
medium mixed salad with
  tomato, lettuce, and
  cucumber and 1 tbs light
  dressing (or *Carottes Vichy/*
  Sliced Carrots with Parsley,
  page 257)
½ cup plain low-fat yogurt
beverage

DINNER
4 oz flounder or other white fish
  with ¾ cup cooked mixed
  vegetables, green beans, or
  spinach (or *Pot-au-Feu de la
  Mer/*Fish Stew with Herbs,
  page 309)
1 orange
beverage

DAY THREE

BREAKFAST
1 oz low-fat cheese
½ cup orange juice
beverage

LUNCH
4 oz broiled or cold skinless
  chicken breast with ¾ cup
  cooked tomatoes (or *Poulet
  Basquaise/*Stewed Chicken
  Basque Style, page 280)
1 piece fruit
beverage

DINNER
4 oz grilled veal chop
¾ cup cooked green beans or
    Brussels sprouts
½ cup low-fat cottage cheese
beverage

DAY FOUR

BREAKFAST
½ cup plain low-fat yogurt
½ cup orange juice
beverage

LUNCH
4 oz lean cold cuts: any
    combination of turkey, roast
    beef, or ham with medium
    mixed salad and 1 tbs light
    dressing (or *Courgettes Farcies/*
    Stuffed Zucchini, page 260)
2 oz low-fat cheese
beverage

DINNER
large mixed salad of tomatoes
    and cucumber with 1 tbs
    light dressing
4 oz sole or other white fish
½ cup low-fat cottage cheese
1 apple
beverage

DAY FIVE

BREAKFAST
1 egg, any style
½ cup orange juice
½ plain low-fat yogurt
beverage

LUNCH
medium chef's salad (1 slice of
    chicken, turkey, lean ham,
    tomato, salad greens) with
    1 tbs light dressing
½ cup plain low-fat yogurt
beverage

DINNER
4 oz lean pork
1½ cups steamed broccoli,
    cauliflower, or cabbage
2 oz low-fat cheese
1 piece fruit
beverage

DAY SIX

BREAKFAST
½ cup plain low-fat yogurt with
    1 piece chopped fruit
beverage

LUNCH
3–4 oz individual can of water-
    packed tuna
1 large tomato, 1½ cups raw
    celery, or ¾ small cucumber
½ cup sherbet flavored with
    artificial sweetener
beverage

DINNER
5 oz lamb with 1 cup cooked
    squash or broccoli (or *Sauté de
    Veau aux Petits Légumes*/Sautéed
    Veal with Vegetables,
    page 268)
½ cup low-fat cottage cheese
beverage

DAY SEVEN

BREAKFAST
½ cup plain low-fat yogurt
½ cup unsweetened grapefruit
    juice
beverage

LUNCH
large mixed salad with 1 tbs
    light dressing
4 oz cold lean meat
1 oz low-fat cheese
beverage

DINNER
½ cup low-fat cottage cheese
    with chives and cucumber
    slices
4 oz broiled skinless turkey
¾ cup cooked green beans,
    spinach, or zucchini
1 piece fruit
beverage

DAY EIGHT

BREAKFAST
½ cup low-fat cottage cheese
apricots, 2 medium fresh or 4
    halves canned in own juice
beverage

LUNCH
large mixed salad with 1 tbs
    light dressing
4 oz broiled hamburger with
    1 slice low-fat cheese
½ cup plain low-fat yogurt
beverage

DINNER
medium green salad with 1 tbs
    light dressing
4 oz broiled lean veal chop
¾ cup cooked green beans,
    Brussels sprouts, or broccoli
1 piece fruit
beverage

DAY NINE

BREAKFAST
1 cup plain low-fat yogurt
beverage

LUNCH
2 eggs, any style, with 2 medium
    baked tomatoes (or *Piperade/*
    Scrambled Eggs with
    Tomatoes and Sweet Peppers,
    page 286)
½ cup low-fat cottage cheese
    with 1 piece chopped fruit
beverage

DINNER
6 oz tomato or vegetable juice
4 oz filet of sole or other white
    fish
½ cup cooked spinach, zucchini,
    or carrots
1 piece fruit
beverage

DAY TEN

BREAKFAST
½ cup low-fat cottage cheese
½ cup orange juice
beverage

LUNCH
large chef's salad (1 slice of
    chicken, turkey, lean ham,
    tomato, salad greens) with
    1 tbs light dressing
beverage

DINNER
medium green salad with
    2 medium tomatoes, 1 oz
    sliced hard cheese and 1 tbs
    light dressing
4 oz broiled lean steak
½ cup plain low-fat yogurt with
    1 piece chopped fruit
beverage

DAY ELEVEN

BREAKFAST
½ cup plain low-fat yogurt
½ cup orange juice
beverage

LUNCH
4 oz lean hamburger
¾ cup cooked green peas or
    carrots or medium green
    salad with 1 tbs light dressing
½ cup low-fat cottage cheese
beverage

DINNER
medium green salad with 1 tbs
    light dressing
4 oz chicken breast with ¾ cup
    steamed mixed vegetables and
    1 oz grated low-fat cheese
1 peach
beverage

DAY TWELVE

BREAKFAST
2 slices low-fat cheese
½ cup unsweetened grapefruit
    juice
beverage

LUNCH
3–4 oz individual can of water-
    packed tuna or salmon with
    medium mixed salad and
    1 tbs light dressing (or *Moules
    Marinières*/Steamed Mussels,
    page 293)
½ cup plain low-fat yogurt
beverage

DINNER
1 cup clear broth (not chunky or
    creamy soup)
medium green salad with
    1 medium tomato plus 1 tbs
    light dressing
4 oz broiled lean steak with
    ¾ cup cooked mushrooms,
    tomatoes, or peppers

½ cup low-fat cottage cheese
with 1 piece chopped fruit
beverage

DAY THIRTEEN

BREAKFAST
½ cup low-fat cottage cheese
beverage

LUNCH
4 oz cold skinless chicken (or
    Émincé de Veau à la Sauge/Veal
    Cutlets with Sage, page 269)
¾ cup cooked zucchini or
    mixed vegetables topped with
    1 oz grated low-fat cheese
1 piece fruit
beverage

DINNER
medium mixed salad with 1 tbs
    light dressing (or *Salade
    Maraîchère*/Raw Vegetable
    Salad, page 244)
4 oz broiled sole or other white
    fish
12 steamed asparagus tips or
    ¾ cup cooked squash or
    mixed vegetables
½ cup plain low-fat yogurt with
    1 piece chopped fruit
beverage

DAY FOURTEEN

BREAKFAST
½ cup plain low-fat yogurt
½ cup orange juice
beverage

LUNCH
4 oz turkey breast
¾ cup cooked broccoli or
    spinach
1 oz low-fat cheese
beverage

DINNER
medium green salad with 1 tbs
    light dressing
4 oz lean ham
¾ cup cooked tomatoes (or
    ¾ cup *Ratatouille*/Stewed
    Vegetables Mediterranean
    Style, page 263)
½ cup low-fat cottage cheese
    with 1 piece chopped fruit
beverage

The Weight Loss Program: Stage Two
The Chef's Menu

Here again is the gourmet side of life—our Chef's Menu. If you find
it easier to follow the summary or standard diet plans, try to incorporate a few of the chef's recipes into the week anyway. The more
delicious the diet, the easier it will be to stay on.

These recipes can be found on the pages listed in the menu plans.

DAY ONE

BREAKFAST
½ cup plain low-fat yogurt or
    low-fat cottage cheese
½ cup unsweetened grapefruit
    juice
beverage

LUNCH
Omelette Soufflée (Fluffy Omelet),
    page 288
1 cup plain low-fat yogurt
beverage

DINNER
medium green salad with
    2 medium tomatoes with
    1 tbs light dressing
*Filet de Sole à la Purée de
    Concombre* (Filet of Sole with
    Cucumber Purée), page 301

Aspic de Fruits Frais aux Saveurs
Exotiques (Fresh Fruit Aspic
with Exotic Flavors),
page 315
beverage

DAY TWO

BREAKFAST

½ cup plain low-fat yogurt or
low-fat cottage cheese with
1 piece chopped fruit
beverage

LUNCH

Asperges aux Champignons en Duo
(Duet of Asparagus and
Mushrooms), page 255
*Jambonnette de Volaille au Parfum de
Truffes* (Chicken Flavored with
Truffles), page 275
¾ cup purée of green beans
beverage

DINNER

medium green salad with 1 oz
diced hard low-fat cheese and
1 tbs light dressing
Courgettes Farcies (Stuffed
Zucchini), page 260
Yogourt Glacé au Coulis de Kiwi
(Frozen Yogurt with Kiwi
Sauce), page 313
beverage

DAY THREE

BREAKFAST

½ cup plain low-fat yogurt or
low-fat cottage cheese
½ cup unsweetened pineapple
juice
beverage

LUNCH

Salade Marignan (Mixed Vegetable
Salad), page 245
1 slice lean ham
1 oz low-fat cheese
beverage

DINNER
6 oz tomato or vegetable juice
1 cup low-fat cottage cheese
    with herbs and cucumber
    slices
shish kebab of 4 oz fish (red
    snapper, sole, etc.), tomatoes,
    peppers on a skewer
Pommes Surprises au Four (Baked
    Apple Surprise), page 310
beverage

DAY FOUR

BREAKFAST
½ cup plain low-fat yogurt or
    low-fat cottage cheese
½ cup unsweetened grapefruit
    juice
beverage

LUNCH
medium chef's salad (greens,
    tomatoes, 2 oz cold chicken,
    hard-boiled egg, 2 slices of
    low-fat cheese, shredded)
    with 1 tbs light dressing
1 pear
beverage

DINNER
Soufflé de Brocolis aux Deux Épices
    (Broccoli Soufflé with Two
    Spices), page 256
2 thin slices of turkey
½ cup plain low-fat yogurt
beverage

DAY FIVE

BREAKFAST

1 cup plain low-fat yogurt or
low-fat cottage cheese
½ cup grapefruit juice
beverage

LUNCH

Gaspacho de Tomates (Tomato
Gazpacho), page 243
*Oeufs Durs ou Pochés Florentines aux
Épinards* (Hard-Cooked or
Poached Eggs with Spinach),
page 287
beverage

DINNER

large green salad with 2 medium
tomatoes, 1 oz diced hard
low-fat cheese, and 1 tbs light
dressing
mixed grill (assorted shish
kebabs—4 oz of fish, turkey,
chicken, or beef and tomatoes
and peppers on a skewer)
1 piece fruit
beverage

DAY SIX

BREAKFAST

½ cup plain low-fat yogurt or
low-fat cottage cheese
½ cup orange juice
beverage

LUNCH

medium green salad with
2 medium tomatoes and
1 tbs light dressing
*Gratin de St. Jacques à l'Effiloché
d'Endives* (Scallops Gratin with
a Fringe of Endive), page 294
½ cup low-fat cottage cheese
beverage

DINNER

medium watercress salad with
1 oz diced hard low-fat
cheese and 1 tbs light
dressing

DINNER *(cont'd)*
4 oz grilled veal chop
Soupe de Fraises au Champagne
   (Strawberries in Champagne),
   page 312
beverage

DAY SEVEN

BREAKFAST
½ cup plain low-fat yogurt or
   low-fat cottage cheese
beverage

LUNCH
4 oz grilled hamburger with
   1 slice low-fat cheese
1 cup cooked green peas
1 cup plain low-fat yogurt with
   1 piece chopped fruit
beverage

DINNER
Truite au Sel (Trout in Salt),
   page 304
1 cup mixed vegetables
Mousse au Chocolat Noir Allégé
   (Low-Calorie Dark Chocolate
   Mousse), page 316
beverage

DAY EIGHT

BREAKFAST
½ cup plain low-fat yogurt or
   low-fat cottage cheese
½ cup unsweetened pineapple
   juice
beverage

LUNCH
1 cup cooked leeks with lemon
   sauce
2 hard-boiled eggs with low-
   calorie dressing
2 slices low-fat cheese
beverage

DINNER
Courgettes aux Crevettes Roses
   (Zucchini with Pink Shrimp),
   page 262

4 oz roast chicken
Brochettes de Fruits en Papillottes
  (Fruit Skewers), page 316
beverage

DAY NINE

BREAKFAST
½ cup plain low-fat yogurt or
  low-fat cottage cheese with
  1 piece chopped fruit
beverage

LUNCH
large mixed salad (tomato,
  greens, cucumber, and 1 oz
  diced hard low-fat cheese)
  with 1 tbs light dressing
Sole aux Raisins (Sole with
  Grapes), page 302
beverage

DINNER
large green bean salad with 1 tbs
  light dressing
4 oz cold roast beef
½ cup plain low-fat yogurt
beverage

DAY TEN

BREAKFAST
½ cup plain low-fat yogurt or
  low-fat cottage cheese
1 soft-boiled egg
beverage

LUNCH
¾ cup raw mushrooms with
  lemon juice
Fondant de Volaille au Whisky
  (Chicken Salad with Whiskey
  Dressing), page 282
1 cup plain low-fat yogurt with
  1 piece chopped fruit
beverage

DINNER
6 oz tomato or vegetable juice
Petit Homard à la Vapeur (Steamed
   Baby Lobster with
   Vegetables), page 305
Pétales de Kiwi au Jus de Fraises
   (Kiwi Petals with Strawberry
   Purée), page 313
beverage

DAY ELEVEN

BREAKFAST
½ cup plain low-fat yogurt or
   low-fat cottage cheese
½ cup grapefruit juice
beverage

LUNCH
6 oz red snapper baked in foil
1 cup mixed vegetables
1 cup low-fat cottage cheese
beverage

DINNER
*Pilon de Volaille Cuit au Senteur
   d'Estragon* (Tarragon-Flavored
   Chicken), page 276
½ cup cauliflower purée
1 piece fruit
beverage

DAY TWELVE

BREAKFAST
1 cup plain low-fat yogurt or
   low-fat cottage cheese
1 piece fruit
beverage

LUNCH
large green salad with 1 tbs light
   dressing
4 oz total assortment of cold
   meats (1 oz ham, 1 oz roast
   beef, 1 oz roast pork, 1 oz
   turkey)
Mousse aux Deux Fruits (Two-Fruit
   Mousse), page 314
beverage

DINNER

4 oz poached haddock or sole
1 cup cooked spinach or 2 cups
raw spinach with 1 tbs light
dressing
1 oz low-fat cheese
beverage

DAY THIRTEEN

BREAKFAST
1 cup low-fat cottage cheese
beverage

LUNCH
Cocktail de Crevettes au Soja
(Shrimp Salad with Sprouts),
page 299
1 cup plain low-fat yogurt with
1 piece chopped fruit
beverage

DINNER
6 oz tomato or vegetable juice
Filet de Boeuf Grand-Mère (Old-
Fashioned Filet of Beef),
page 265
*Aspic de Fruits Frais aux Saveurs
Exotiques* (Fresh Fruit Aspic
with Exotic Flavors),
page 315
beverage

DAY FOURTEEN

BREAKFAST
½ cup plain low-fat yogurt or
   low-fat cottage cheese
½ cup orange juice
beverage

LUNCH
Poulet Pané au Sésame (Breaded
   Chicken with Sesame Seeds),
   page 278
1 cup steamed cauliflower
¾ cup strawberries
beverage

DINNER
6 large grilled shrimp
1 cup steamed mixed vegetables
½ cup plain low-fat yogurt
beverage

PART FOUR

❖

The Paris Diet:
The Adjustment Program

STAGE ONE *(2 weeks)*
STAGE TWO *(2-4 weeks)*

———— ❖ ————

CHAPTER 9

The Adjustment Program:
Stages One and Two

*F*or those of you who have followed our program from the beginning—the life-dieters—this should be a red-letter day. You have now reached the third phase of the Paris Diet: the Adjustment Program. At this point, you've probably lost a significant amount of weight. Now, the program will carefully increase your food intake so that you won't gain any back even though you'll be eating more than you did before. Follow Stage One for two weeks, then go to Stage Two for another two weeks; however, to "set" your new weight, one month at Stage Two is better.

The calorie intake for Stage One and Stage Two of the Adjustment Program is identical to that of Stage One and Stage Two of the Preparation Program. We will refer you to the appropriate pages in Chapters 5 and 6 to avoid repeating the menus here.

One note of caution to life-dieters: If you don't want to find yourself back in that old cycle of constant dieting or eating too little only to gain weight the minute you indulge, stick to this program. Don't fool yourself into thinking it's better for you to continue to restrict your food intake. The only way you'll keep the weight off permanently is to eat a normal amount of food. That's the basis of the entire Paris Diet. Life-dieters must gradually work their way up to eating 1,600, 1,800, or even 2,000 calories each day.

Some of you will be starting the program with this stage. You are people who:

1. are large or
2. are average to healthy eaters (1,500 to 2,400 calories daily) and have twenty pounds or less to lose or

3. are hearty eaters (2,500 to 3,000 calories daily) and have twenty pounds or more to lose or

4. are heavy eaters (over 3,000 calories daily) and have twenty pounds or more to lose—you will start with two weeks at Stage Two; you should skip Stage One.

If you start with the Adjustment Program and go through to the Maintenance Program without losing all the weight you want, stay at the 2,000-calorie level for one month, and then start the program over using the following schedule:

Weight Loss Program: Stage One	2 weeks	(Chapter 7)
Weight Loss Program: Stage Two	2 weeks	(Chapter 8)
Preparation Program: Stage One	2 weeks	(Chapter 5)
Preparation Program: Stage Two	2 weeks	(Chapter 6)
Maintenance Program: Stage One	2 weeks	(Chapter 10)
Maintenance Program: Stage Two	2 weeks	(Chapter 11)
Maintenance Program: Stage Three	2 weeks	(Chapter 11)

Make sure to exercise during the Adjustment Program. This helps to firm, tone, and strengthen your body. Our exercise program, which perfectly complements the stages of the Paris Diet, is detailed in Chapter 12.

Whether you are starting the program with the Adjustment Program or marking it as step three, use the guidelines and suggestions for the Preparation Program included in Chapters 5 and 6. They will tell you how to cook and prepare your food, how to use dressings, and what to do in every eating situation. In addition, tables of prohibited and authorized foods that appear on pages 67–70 should be used for both levels of the Adjustment Program.

You're ready to start the Adjustment Program. The Paris Diet offers you three menu choices for each stage in this program. You can follow the Summary Plan, which tells you the basic foods and amounts you have to eat. Use the exchange (equivalency) tables that appear on pages 70–73.

You might follow the Standard Diet, which gives you two weeks of simple, yet appetizing meals. If you love fine food, try our Chef's Menu, which comes from some of the finest professional cooks in Paris!

Finally, you could combine them. For example, you might follow the Summary Plan for busy days or at a restaurant; the Standard Diet for evening meals or lazy days around the house; and the Chef's Menu for weekends or whenever you want gourmet meals that are quick and easy to prepare.

For those using the Adjustment Program as phase three, you will now find that food can be hearty and delicious without being fattening. For those who are starting the program here, we can promise that you'll lose all the weight you want, you won't feel hungry, and you'll be able to eat normally again, for the rest of your life, without gaining back an ounce!

The Adjustment Program: Stage One
Summary for Easy Reference

On this stage of the diet, you will eat certain basic foods each day. If you don't want to follow the Standard Diet or Chef's Menu, use this summary for any or all of the days. You might choose to follow the Chef's Menu on the weekends, but on a busy Monday, substitute the simple foods listed below.

If you want to have even more choice in the selection of your daily meals, refer to the exchange tables on pages 70–73 to find out which foods are the exact equivalents of the ones below. If you do make a substitution, be sure to use the specific quantities in the tables. For example, 1 cup of plain low-fat yogurt is equal to 1⅓ cups of skim milk. You could have either and adhere to the diet. However, if you drink 2 cups of skim milk in place of 1 cup of yogurt, you'd be consuming too many calories.

You might want to photocopy the summary page to have it with you when you're away from home, so you'll never be in doubt about how much and what to eat.

The Adjustment Program: Stage One

Summary Plan

BREAKFAST

½ cup plain low-fat yogurt
2 slices of bread (any type of regular white or whole wheat
   with no fruit or honey added)
½ cup fruit juice (if you eliminate one fruit serving
   from another meal)
1 pat butter or margarine
beverage

LUNCH

small green salad or 3 oz raw vegetables with 1 tbs light dressing
4 oz lean meat or skinless poultry or fish, cooked without fat
¾ cup boiled or steamed vegetables, cooked without fat
1 slice or 1 oz low-fat cheese
1 medium-size piece or ½ cup fruit
beverage

DINNER

4 oz lean meat or skinless poultry or fish, cooked without fat
¾ cup boiled or steamed vegetables, cooked without fat
½ cup plain low-fat yogurt
1 medium-size piece or ½ cup fruit
beverage

For Men

Since men have more muscle mass and therefore slightly higher
protein needs than women, men must add one of the following:

   2 whites of eggs (no yolks), hard boiled, chopped into salads, or
   ¼ cup low-fat cottage cheese, or
   ½ cup plain low-fat yogurt, or
   1 slice of ham or turkey or roast beef

These extra foods can be eaten at any point in the day and should
be added to the Summary Plan, Standard Diet, and Chef's Menu.

The Adjustment Program: Stage One

Since the Adjustment Program has the identical caloric intake as the Preparation Program, there is no need to repeat the specific menus. This list will help you to find the menus for Stage One of the Adjustment Program:

The Adjustment Program: Stage Two

Summary for Easy Reference

On this stage of the diet, you will eat certain basic foods each day. If you don't want to follow the Standard Diet or Chef's menu, use this summary for any and all of the days. You might choose to follow the Chef's Menu on the weekends, but on a busy Monday, substitute the simple foods listed below.

If you want to have even more choice in the selection of your daily meals, refer to the exchange tables on page 70 to find out which foods are the exact equivalents of the ones below. If you do make a substitution, use the exact quantities in the tables. For example, 1 cup of plain low-fat yogurt is equal to 1⅓ cups of skim milk. You could have either and adhere to the diet. However, if you drink 2 cups of skim milk in place of 1 cup of yogurt, you'd be consuming too many calories.

You might want to photocopy the summary page to have it with you when you're away from home, so you'll never be in doubt about how much and what to eat.

The Adjustment Program: Stage Two

Summary Plan

BREAKFAST

½ cup plain low-fat yogurt or ½ cup low-fat cottage cheese
½ cup unsweetened fruit juice or piece of fruit (can be saved for
   dessert at lunch or dinner)
2 slices plain bread or toast (any type) with 2 pats butter or
   margarine
beverage

LUNCH

medium green salad with 1 tbs oil or regular salad dressing
¾ cup cooked or 1½ cups raw vegetables (boiled or steamed
   without oil or fat)
4 oz meat or fish (cooked without oil or fat—baked, broiled,
   steamed, or grilled only)
1 oz or 1 slice low-fat cheese
1 slice plain bread or toast (any type) or 4 plain crackers
1 medium-size piece or ½ cup chopped fruit
beverage

DINNER

medium green salad with 1 tbs light dressing (see our recipes)
4 oz lean meat or fish (cooked without oil or fat—baked, broiled,
   steamed or grilled only)
2 medium potatoes or starch equivalents (see exchange tables),
   cooked without fat
½ cup plain low-fat yogurt or ½ cup low-fat cottage cheese
beverage

For Men

Since men have more muscle mass and therefore slightly higher
protein needs than women, men must add one of the following:

2 whites of eggs (no yolks), hard boiled, chopped into salads, or
¼ cup low fat cottage cheese, or

½ cup plain low-fat yogurt, or
1 slice of ham or turkey or roast beef

The Adjustment Program: Stage Two

Since the Adjustment Program has the identical caloric intake as the Preparation Program, there is no need to repeat the specific menus. This list will help you to find the menus for Stage Two of the Adjustment Program:

Now you are ready to move on to the Maintenance Program—a way to eat for the rest of your life that will keep you healthy *and* slim.

PART FIVE

❖

The Paris Diet:
The
Maintenance
Program

STAGE ONE   *(2–4 weeks)*
STAGE TWO   *(2–4 weeks)*
STAGE THREE   *(2–4 weeks)*

CHAPTER 10

The Maintenance Program:
Stage One

A 1,600-calorie diet is the first stage in the Maintenance Program—the way you'll be eating for the rest of your life. You now have reached the point where you are eating normally but healthier. If you're a heavy eater, you're losing weight as well. Light eaters and life-dieters won't believe how much food they can safely enjoy without gaining an ounce.

Although the success of the Maintenance Program depends largely on how carefully and regularly you follow it, the French are not known to be disciplinarians when it comes to sensual pleasure. We don't measure a balanced diet on a day-to-day basis, but rather by the week. You are now allowed an occasional—but we mean occasional—lapse. If you have to taste that special candy bar, go ahead. Just watch your caloric intake for the next few days.

Of course, the success of any diet is its feasibility. If it's too hard to follow, you are likely to abandon it. The Paris Diet has taken this into consideration and has made its food as appetizing as possible. But you won't be able to eat all the high-calorie foods you might have consumed in the past. Don't lose your momentum; the splendid effort you've made for all this time will soon have its major benefit.

The basis of the 1,600-calorie Maintenance Program is the 1,200 calorie diet. Just as you added an extra helping of starch to raise it to 1,400 calories, you will now include even more food to bring your daily intake up to 1,600 calories. What you add to the 1,600-calorie program is a controlled level of fat, which is needed for a balanced diet.

Follow this plan for two weeks (or for best results, a month).

There is all sorts of good news during this phase of the diet. For convenience, you can now have a frozen prepared diet meal if you choose. If you don't want to add fat to your meals, you can take in the extra food in some self-indulgent ways:

If you feel like drinking an alcoholic beverage, you can now do it. For cocktails, you can have any one of the following:

2 glasses of champagne plus 15 pistachios or 6 salted nuts
1 Tom Collins
1 whiskey sour plus 10 medium olives
1 martini cocktail plus 8 roasted peanuts
1 Manhattan cocktail plus 10 pistachios
1 gin, rum, vodka, or whiskey (2 fl oz) plus 6–8 almonds or peanuts

If you're French or just feel like it, you can have instead, for lunch or dinner:

2 ½ glasses of white or red wine

If you plan to drink, substitute a low-fat dressing for any oils or fats in the menu.

If you want to eat French fries, a pizza, a hamburger, or a juicy sandwich, do it—but no more than twice a week (fries should be eaten only once a week). You can have these meals with a salad, with a tablespoon of light dressing.

If you want ice cream or pastry, go ahead, but no more than once a week. If you choose to indulge your sweet tooth, don't eat any starchy foods on the same or following day; eat only vegetables with the main meals.

NOTE: Don't eat French fries, ice cream, and have a drink all on the same day.

The following pages list the prohibited and authorized foods for the 1,600-calorie Maintenance Program. For the rest of the Maintenance Program, there are no food restrictions—just your own judgment about eating better and having the right kinds of meals.

You also will find a list of food exchanges for the 1,600- 1,800-, and 2,000-calorie diets in the pages that follow. Use these with the Summary Plan, or to vary the foods in the Standard Diet and Chef's Menu.

The Maintenance Program: Stage One

Prohibited Foods

For easier selection, here is a list of foods you cannot eat during Stage One of the Maintenance Program (1,600 calories). You can see that it is essentially the same as the list for the Adjustment Program (1,200 and 1,400 calories), except that alcohol is now permitted. When you move on to Stage Two and (if appropriate) Stage Three of this program, there are no restricted foods.

Sometimes a prohibited food is included in the menus that follow. We do this to give your mind and taste buds a treat, but don't add one yourself. Follow the meal plans carefully, and only add indulgences where indicated.

SUGAR AND SWEETENED PRODUCTS
sugar, honey, jams, "diet jams", jellies, cookies, pastries, ice cream, sherbet, candies, chocolate, chocolate-flavored drinks, chewing gum with sugar, sorbitol or xylitol (sweeteners that contain significant calories), yogurt or other daily products with flavorings or fruit added, candied fruit, fruit in syrup, canned fruit compote, dried fruits (apricots, dates, figs, prunes, raisins, etc.), syrups, canned or bottled fruit juices, soda, cereal bars

FATTY FOODS (to be eaten no more than once per week)
sauces, fried foods, French fries, potato chips, doughnuts, pizza, quiche, avocados, and anything cooked with oil or fat

Deli Meats: pâté, salami, bologna, frankfurters, sausages, wursts, corned beef, pastrami, tongue

Fatty Meats: pork, mutton, lamb, duck, goose, venison, fatty cuts of beef (like filet mignon or chuck)

Fish and Shellfish: eel, lamprey, breaded fish, fish canned in oil, clams, oysters

Dairy Foods with high fat content: cheeses with greater than 50 percent fat content: Roquefort, Gorgonzola, bleu, Brillat-Savarin, St.

Andre, Bour&ault, Caprice des Dieux, regular and goat cheeses with
boosted cream content, creamed cheese, creamed Swiss cheese; regular or creamed cottage cheese or yogurt, whole milk
   Nuts: almonds, peanuts, hazelnuts, walnuts, cashews, pine nuts,
brazils, etc.

Authorized Foods

Here's what you can eat at the Stage One maintenance level. Try our
special sauces and dressings to add bulk and flavoring to your meals.
Shrimp Parfaits, Zucchini with Meat Stuffing, Tandoori Chicken, and
Baked Apple Surprise are just some of the dishes you and your family
can enjoy.

LEAN, TRIMMED MEATS
beef, veal, chicken (all poultry to be eaten without skin), pheasant,
turkey and chicken cutlets, roast turkey, rabbit, lean lamb; very lean
roast pork, filet of pork or pork chop can be eaten once a week

LEAN FISH
cod, haddock, pollack, lemon sole, sole, bass, whiting, ray, red mullet,
red snapper, turbot

FATTY FISH
shad, anchovies, carp, herring, lake trout, mackerel, sardines, salmon,
tuna, all packed in water (no oil)
         EAT FISH, LEAN OR FATTY, SEVERAL TIMES EACH WEEK

FRESH FRUITS AND VEGETABLES

STARCHES
breads, flaky rolls, crackers, melba toast, breadsticks, matzo, cocktail
snack crackers, cereals, pasta, rice, semolina, potatoes, dried legumes
(white beans, lentils, split peas, chick peas)

ALCOHOLIC BEVERAGES (as indicated on page 182)

DAIRY FOODS, LOW-FAT
cheeses with less than 50 percent fat content: low-fat Camembert,
Comte, Coulommiers, low-fat Bries, Gruyère, Port du Salut, Edam,

Gouda, Mimolette, Cheshire, low-fat goat cheese, Roblochon, Saint Nectaire, Tomme; 1–2 percent low-fat plain yogurt and low-fat plain cottage cheese.

The Maintenance Program: Exchange (Equivalency) Tables

The following tables list foods in different categories that are approximately the same, calorie-wise, as other foods. You should use them in two ways. First, these tables will form the basis of the Summary Plan. If lunch calls for ½ cup of cooked vegetables, just look at the vegetable exchange list to see which ones you can choose from.

You can also use these lists to vary your diet if you are following the set menu plans. This is advisable since boredom sabotages any regimen. Simply pick a food from the lists that equals the one in the plan and substitute it. Make sure you use the quantity listed or it won't be equal in caloric value to the food for which it's being exchanged. For example, if you don't feel like having ½ cup of beets, exchange it for 6 ounces of tomato juice—not 4 or 8 ounces but 6 ounces.

Not all foods in the menu plans will have exchanges.

Each one of the foods contained within a numbered list is equal to all others in that list. You can also choose to make two exchanges: For instance, if you want to eat 1 apple, you can either exchange it for 1 small banana, or for 10 cherries plus ½ cup of orange juice. It's up to you.

If the menu calls for 4 ounces of beef, and the exchange table lists beef in quantities of 1 ounce, remember to multiply all the other quantities in the list by 4 if you are exchanging for the beef. In other words, since 1 ounce of beef equals 1 slice of low-fat cheese, 4 ounces of beef would be equal to 4 slices of low-fat cheese.

I. Vegetable Exchanges (for ½ cup cooked or 1 cup raw)

asparagus	beets
beans (green or wax)	broccoli
bean sprouts	Brussels sprouts

cabbage (all kinds)
carrots
catsup, 2 tablespoons
cauliflower
celery
cucumber
eggplant
leafy greens (all kinds)
mushrooms

okra
onion
pepper (red or green)
rutabaga
sauerkraut
squash, summer
tomato
tomato or vegetable juice,
    6 ounces

II. Fruit Exchanges
FRUITS
apple, ½ medium
applesauce, ½ cup
apricots, dried, 4 halves
apricots, fresh, 2 medium
banana, ½ small
blueberries, ½ cup
cantaloupe, (6-inch diameter)
    ¼ medium
cherries, 10 large
dates, 2
figs, dried, 1 small
fruit cocktail, canned, ½ cup
grapefruit, ½ small
grapes, 15 small
JUICES
apple, pineapple,
grapefruit, orange, ½ cup

honeydew melon (7-inch
    diameter), ⅓
mango, ½ small
nectarine, 1 small
orange, 1 small
papaya, ⅓ medium
peach, 1 medium
pear, 1 small
pineapple, ½ cup
prunes, dried, 2
raisins, 2 tablespoons
strawberries, ¾ cup
tangerine, 1 large
watermelon, 1 cup cubed

grape, prune, ¼ cup

III. Starch Exchanges (cooked servings)
BREADS
bagel, ½
bun for hamburger or
    hot dog, ½
cornbread (1½-inch diameter),
    1 cube

dinner roll (2-inch diameter), 1
English muffin, ½
plain bread (no honey or fruit
    added), 1 slice
tortilla (6-inch diameter), 1

CRACKERS
graham (2½-inch square), 2
matzo (4 by 6 inches), ½
melba toast, 4
oyster crackers (½ cup), 20

pretzels, 8 rings
rye krisps, 3
saltines, 5

CEREALS
bran, 5 tablespoons
dry flakes, ⅔ cup
dry puffed, 1½ cups
hot cereal such as oatmeal,
    farina, ½ cup

pastas, ½ cup
rice, ½ cup
wheat germ, 2 tablespoons

STARCHY VEGETABLES
beans or peas (plain),
    ½ cup
corn, ⅓ cup or ½ medium ear
parsnips, ⅔ cup

potatoes, white, 1 small or
    ½ cup
potatoes, sweet or yams, ¼ cup
pumpkin, ¾ cup
squash, winter, ½ cup

DESSERTS
angel cake, 1½ inch square

fat-free sherbet, 4 ounces

IV. Protein Exchanges (cooked weight)
beef, dried, chipped, 1 ounce
beef, lamb, pork, veal (lean
    only), 1 ounce
cheese, hard, ½ ounce
cheese, low fat, 1 ounce or
    1 slice
cottage cheese, plain, low fat,
    ¼ cup*
egg, 1 medium

fish, 1 ounce
lobster, 1 small tail
oysters, clams, shrimps,
    5 medium
peanut butter, 2 teaspoons
poultry, without skin, 1 ounce
salmon, pink, canned, ¼ cup
tuna, packed in water, ¼ cup

* Note: Cheeses contain good amounts of protein and calcium; therefore, they are listed in two tables and can be used either as an exchange for a protein-rich food or as an exchange for a dairy food.

V. *Dairy Exchanges*

cheese, hard, ½ ounce
cheese, low fat, 1 ounce or
    1 slice
cottage cheese, plain, low fat,
    ¼ cup

milk, 1% fat, ½ cup
milk, skim, ⅔ cup
yogurt, plain, low fat, ½ cup

VI. *Fat Exchanges*

avocado (4-inch diameter), ⅛
bacon, crisp, 1 slice
butter or margarine, 1 pat
French dressing, 1 tablespoon
mayonnaise, 2 teaspoons
oil, 2 teaspoons (all kinds)

olives, 5 small
peanuts, 10
Roquefort dressing, 1 tablespoon
Thousand Island dressing,
    1 tablespoon
walnuts, 6 small

The Maintenance Program: Stage One

Summary for Easy Reference

On this stage of the diet, you will eat certain basic foods each day. If you don't want to follow the Standard Diet or Chef's Menu, use this summary for any or all of the days. You might choose to follow the Chef's Menu on the weekends, but on a busy Monday, substitute the simple foods listed below.

If you want to have even more choice in the selection of your daily meals, refer to the exchange tables to find out which foods are the exact equivalents of the ones below. If you do make a substitution, use the exact quantities in the tables. For example, 1 cup of plain low-fat yogurt is equal to 1⅓ cups of skim milk. You could have either and adhere to the diet. However, if you drink 2 cups of skim milk in place of 1 cup of yogurt, you'd be consuming too many calories.

You might want to photocopy the summary page to have it with you when you're away from home, so you'll never be in doubt about how much and what to eat.

The Maintenance Program: Stage One

Summary Plan

BREAKFAST

3 slices plain bread (any type) with 2 pats butter or margarine; or
1 cup any cereal with ½ cup skim milk, no sugar, artificial
sweetener permitted; or 1 English muffin with 1 pat butter or
margarine
½ cup plain low-fat yogurt or ½ cup low-fat cottage cheese
½ cup unsweetened fruit juice or 1 piece of fruit (can be saved for
dessert at lunch or dinner)
beverage

LUNCH

medium green salad with 1 tbs oil or regular salad dressing
1 low-calorie prepared meal, or 1 cup cooked vegetables
(boiled or steamed without oil or fat) or 2 cups raw vegetables
with 1 pat butter or margarine
4 oz lean meat or fish (cooked without oil or fat—baked, broiled,
steamed, or grilled only)
1 slice or 1 oz low-fat cheese
1 slice plain bread (any type) or 4 plain crackers
1 medium-size piece or ½ cup fruit
beverage

DINNER

medium green salad with 1 tbs oil or regular salad dressing
4 oz lean meat or fish (cooked without oil or fat—baked, broiled,
steamed, or grilled only)
2 medium potatoes or starchy foods (see exchange tables) with 1 pat
butter or margarine
½ cup plain low-fat yogurt or ½ cup low-fat cottage cheese
beverage

For Men

At this calorie level and beyond, men no longer need to raise the amount of protein. Therefore, a husband and wife can now follow the same plan.

The Maintenance Program: Stage One

The Standard Diet

The following menu plan is for one week of the 1,600-calorie Standard Diet. All the meals are simple to find and prepare but very satisfying. If you are going to follow this diet for two weeks or more, just repeat the week, and use the exchange tables to vary your meals.

DAY ONE

BREAKFAST
3 slices plain bread (any type)
    with 2 pats butter or
    margarine
½ cup plain low-fat yogurt
½ cup orange juice
beverage

LUNCH
medium green salad with 1 tbs
    oil or regular salad dressing
4 oz roast chicken or cold
    chicken breast
1 cup cooked green beans,
    mixed vegetables, or zucchini
    with 1 pat butter or
    margarine
1 slice or 1 oz low-fat cheese
1 slice plain bread (any type) or
    4 plain crackers
beverage

DINNER
small mixed salad with 1 tbs oil
    or regular salad dressing
4 oz broiled fish (any kind)
2 medium boiled potatoes with
    1 pat butter or margarine
½ cup plain low-fat yogurt
1 baked apple
beverage

DAY TWO

BREAKFAST
½ cup low-fat cottage cheese
    with 1 piece chopped fruit
1 English muffin with 1 pat
    butter or margarine
beverage

LUNCH
large spinach salad with 1 oz
    diced or sliced low-fat cheese
    and 1 tbs oil or regular salad
    dressing
4 oz lean ham
1 slice plain bread (any type) or
    4 plain crackers
1 piece fruit
beverage

DINNER
large tomato salad with 1 tbs oil
    or regular salad dressing
6 oz lean steak
1½ cups cooked yellow corn
    with 1 pat butter or
    margarine
½ cup plain low-fat yogurt
beverage

DAY THREE

BREAKFAST
1 cup any unsweetened cereal
    with ½ cup skim milk, no
    sugar, artificial sweetener
    permitted
½ cup grapefruit juice
beverage

LUNCH
large mixed salad with 1 tbs oil
    or regular salad dressing
4 oz lean hamburger with 1 slice
    low-fat cheese
1 pear or peach
beverage

DINNER
6 oz tomato or vegetable juice
4 oz trout, sole, or snapper
1 cup cooked rice with 1 pat
    butter or margarine
½ cup plain low-fat yogurt

DINNER (cont'd)
beverage: 2 glasses of wine,
    1 8 oz glass of fruit juice, or
    1 8 oz glass of regular soft drink
    (doesn't have to be diet soft
    drink)

DAY FOUR

BREAKFAST
3 slices plain bread (any type)
    with 2 pats butter or
    margarine
½ cup low-fat cottage cheese
    with 1 piece chopped fruit
beverage

LUNCH
large mixed salad with 1 tbs oil
    or regular salad dressing
1 slice pizza (regular crust)
½ cup orange juice
beverage

DINNER
medium bowl vegetable soup
4 oz chicken or turkey breast
1 cup cooked spinach, tomatoes,
    or broccoli with 1 pat butter
    or margarine
½ cup plain low-fat yogurt with
    1 piece chopped fruit
beverage: 1 beer or 1 6 oz glass
    fruit juice or 1 6 oz glass soft
    drink

DAY FIVE

BREAKFAST
1 English muffin with 1 pat
    butter or margarine
½ cup grapefruit juice
1 slice or 1 oz low-fat cheese
beverage

LUNCH
large mixed salad with 1 tbs oil
    or regular salad dressing
4 oz lean beef, chicken, or
    grilled shrimp
½ cup plain low-fat yogurt
1 piece fruit
beverage

DINNER
6 oz tomato or vegetable juice
1 low-calorie frozen prepared
    meal or 1 cup cooked mixed
    vegetables and 4 oz lean steak
1 slice or 1 oz low-fat cheese
1 slice plain bread (any type) or
    4 plain crackers
1 cup regular ice cream
beverage

DAY SIX

BREAKFAST
2 slices plain bread (any type)
    with 2 pats butter or
    margarine
½ cup plain low-fat yogurt
½ cup grapefruit juice
1 egg with two slices of bacon
beverage

LUNCH
medium green salad with 1 oz
    diced hard low-fat cheese and
    1 tbs oil or regular salad
    dressing
4 oz lean veal or chicken
1 cup cooked carrots, eggplant,
    or spinach with 1 pat butter
    or margarine
beverage

DINNER
medium bowl vegetable soup
4 oz grilled trout or salmon
3 medium mashed potatoes with
    1 pat butter or margarine
½ cup plain low-fat yogurt with
    1 piece chopped fruit
beverage

DAY SEVEN

BREAKFAST
1 cup any unsweetened cereal with ½ cup skim milk, no sugar, artificial sweetener permitted
½ cup orange juice
beverage

LUNCH
medium chef's salad (2 oz turkey, 2 oz roast beef, 1 oz ham, 1 oz low-fat cheese) with 1 tbs oil or regular salad dressing
1 slice plain bread (any type) or 4 plain crackers
½ cup plain low-fat yogurt
beverage

DINNER
medium mixed salad with 1 tbs oil or regular salad dressing
1 low-calorie frozen prepared meal or 1 cup cooked broccoli and 4 oz chicken
½ cup low-fat cottage cheese with 1 piece chopped fruit
beverage

The Maintenance Program: Stage One

Chef's Menu

Here is a week's worth of our Chef's Menus, from some of the greatest cooks in Paris. Although these recipes, listed by page number, are easy to prepare, they are no less delightful and unique than the finest meals served along the banks of the Seine.

DAY ONE

BREAKFAST
3 slices plain bread (any type)
  with 2 pats butter or
  margarine
½ cup plain low-fat yogurt with
  1 piece chopped fruit
beverage

LUNCH
Salade Maraîchère (Raw Vegetable
  Salad), page 244
Émincé de Canard aux Deux Poivres
  (Duck Slivers with Two
  Peppers), page 283
½ cup plain low-fat yogurt
beverage

DINNER
Asperges aux Champignons en Duo
  (Duet of Asparagus and
  Mushrooms), page 255
Filets de Truite aux Petits Légumes
  (Trout Filets with Small
  Vegetables), page 303
1 slice or 1 oz low-fat cheese
1 slice plain bread (any type) or
  4 plain crackers
*Aspic de Fruits Frais aux Saveurs
  Exotiques* (Fresh Fruit Aspic
  with Exotic Flavors),
  page 315
beverage

DAY TWO

BREAKFAST
1 cup any unsweetened cereal
  with ½ cup skim milk, no
  sugar, artificial sweetener
  permitted
1 cup grapefruit juice
beverage

LUNCH
*Gâteau de Carottes au Coulis
  d'Asperges* (Carrot Cakes with
  Asparagus Sauce), page 258
*Pilon de Volaille Cuit aux Senteurs
  d'Estragon* (Tarragon-Flavored
  Chicken), page 276
½ cup plain low-fat yogurt
beverage

DINNER
Gaspacho de Tomates (Tomato
  Gazpacho), page 243
Coquilles St. Jacques à la Provençale
  (Scallops à la Provence),
  page 296
¾ cup cooked spaghetti
Gratin de Fraises à la Cannelle
  (Cinnamon-Flavored
  Strawberries), page 312
beverage

DAY THREE

BREAKFAST
1 English muffin with 1 pat
  butter or margarine
½ cup plain low-fat yogurt
½ cup orange juice
beverage

LUNCH
salade vermeil (salad of radishes,
  mushrooms, and lemon juice)
Saumon Cuit à Basse Température
  (Salmon Cooked at Low
  Temperature), page 292
1 slice or 1 oz low-fat cheese
1 slice plain bread (any type) or
  4 plain crackers
beverage

DINNER
Méli-Mélo de Crevettes Roses aux
  Huîtres (Hodgepodge of Pink
  Shrimp with Oysters),
  page 298
Coeur de Filet de Boeuf aux Épices
  (Beef Filet with Spices),
  page 266
2 medium boiled potatoes with
  1 pat butter or margarine
Mousse aux Deux Fruits (Two-Fruit
  Mousse), page 314
beverage

DAY FOUR

BREAKFAST
3 slices plain bread (any type)
 with 2 pats butter or
 margarine
½ cup plain low-fat yogurt
1 baked apple
beverage

LUNCH
Salade Marignan (Mixed Vegetable
 Salad), page 245
Omelette Soufflée (Fluffy Omelet),
 page 288
½ cup plain low-fat yogurt
beverage

DINNER
small green salad with 1 tbs light
 dressing
Petit Rouget au Fenouil Frais (Red
 Mullet or Snapper with Fresh
 Fennel), page 300
⅘ cup cooked rice with 1 pat
 butter or margarine
1 slice or 1 oz low-fat cheese
 with 4 plain crackers
Pétales de Kiwi au Jus de Fraises
 (Kiwi Petals with Strawberry
 Purée), page 313
beverage: 1½ glasses of wine,
 1 8 oz glass fruit juice, or
 1 8 oz glass regular soft drink

DAY FIVE

BREAKFAST
1 cup any unsweetened cereal
 with ½ cup skim milk, no
 sugar, artificial sweetener
 permitted
½ cup mixed fruit salad
beverage

LUNCH

Salade de Haricots Verts Printanière
(Springtime Green Bean
Salad), page 246

St. Pierre au Citron Vert et au Coco
(Grouper with Lime and
Coconut), page 290

1 cup cooked rice

Mousse au Chocolat Noir Allégé
(Low-Calorie Dark Chocolate
Mousse), page 316

beverage

DINNER

*Aspic de Légumes au Coulis de
Tomates* (Vegetable Aspic with
Tomato Sauce), page 264

Poulet Pané au Sésame (Breaded
Chicken with Sesame Seeds),
page 278

1 cup cooked zucchini,
tomatoes, or green beans

2 slices or 2 oz low-fat cheese
with 4 plain crackers

Brochettes de Fruits en Papillotes
(Fruit Skewers), page 316

beverage

DAY SIX

BREAKFAST

rice pudding, without sugar,
sweetened with pears in their
own juice

beverage

LUNCH

medium salad of cucumber and
tomatoes with 1 tbs oil or
regular salad dressing

Filet de Dinde en Habit-Vert
(Turkey Filet in French
Academy Costume),
page 284

1 cup plain low-fat yogurt with
1 piece chopped fruit

beverage

DINNER

Soufflé de Brocolis aux Deux Épices
(Broccoli Soufflé with Two
Spices), page 256
Rôti de Bar au Varech (Broiled
Bass with Seaweed),
page 289
2 medium potatoes with 1 pat
butter or margarine
Yogourt Glacé au Coulis de Kiwi
(Frozen Yogurt with Kiwi
Sauce), page 313
beverage

DAY SEVEN

BREAKFAST
1 slice or 1 oz low-fat cheese
2 slices plain bread (any type)
with 2 pats butter or
margarine
½ cup grapefruit juice
beverage

LUNCH
medium mixed salad with
steamed leeks and 1 tbs light
dressing
Sole aux Raisins (Sole with
Grapes), page 302
½ cup plain low-fat yogurt with
4 plain crackers
beverage

DINNER
1 Tom Collins (or any medium-
size cocktail), 1 8 oz glass of
tomato or vegetable juice, or
1 8 oz glass of regular soft
drink
large green salad with 1 tbs light
dressing
*Blanc de Volaille aux Spaghetti de
Concombre* (Chicken Breasts
with Cucumber Spaghetti),
page 273

DINNER *(cont'd)*
1 cup cooked spaghetti with
    1 pat butter or margarine
½ cup plain low-fat yogurt
Soupe de Fraises au Champagne
    (Strawberries in Champagne),
    page 312
beverage

CHAPTER 11

The Maintenance Program: Stages Two and Three

At the 1,800- and 2,000-calorie levels, you shouldn't think of the plan as a diet but as maintenance eating. By now, you have a new set of eating habits designed to prevent future weight gain.

For most women, the caloric intake at this stage is much higher than before going on the program. In France, one woman out of five who is overweight eats less than 1,200 calories a day; some eat less than 1,000 calories. In America, the story is very much the same. As you learned in Chapter 3, the Paris Diet changes metabolic efficiency to banish this destructive and restrictive syndrome. And once gone, the best benefit of the program is that it allows women in this category to eat more than they did before and still stay slim.

However, some people have been dieting for so long they can never eat more than 1,600 calories without gaining weight. The way to tell if you're one of these people is to follow Stage One of the Maintenance Program (1,600 calories) for two weeks and then move up to Stage Two (1,800 calories) for a week. If you start regaining weight, cut back to Stage One and stay there. For everyone else, it's best to stay in the 1,800- to 2,000-calorie range for as long as possible.

Eighteen hundred to 2,000 calories are the normal daily intake for women who have not been life-dieters and have not had a weight problem. Now it can be your normal intake as well. It's also the calorie level where you formally stop dieting: There are no more forbidden foods. But even though you can have anything you like, you still must respect the basic rules of proper eating: everything in moderation, everything with variety, or as we say in French, *"De tout, un peu"* (a little of everything).

Because men usually consume far more calories than women, there has never been a report, in tens of thousands of cases observed, of a man putting on weight again when he eats between 1,800 and 2,000 calories per day. In fact, men will end up adding anywhere from 200 to 500 calories more to their daily intake.

The basis of the Maintenance Program is the 1,600-calorie diet (Stage One), which you have just finished—in other words, a varied, protein-rich diet. The variety is up to you. For the first additional 200 and then 400-calorie increase, you can add extra helpings of starch or cook with a little more fat. We have included a Summary Plan that gives you the guidelines for healthy maintenance eating.

You can also design your own maintenance plan. Use the menus from Stage One. To add the extra 200 to 400 calories, you don't have to weigh your food or check the list of equivalents each day. But you will need a bit of imagination, which makes it fun:

1. Continue eating lean meats, but use more fats when you cook.
2. Use real sugar (in moderation) in your coffee, yogurt, or fruit.
3. Eat twice the number of bread or starchy foods that you did on the lower calorie plans if you like.

At this level, you can also enjoy a genuine American breakfast with cereal, toast, jam, and eggs, but no more than twice a week. Don't be afraid of eating a big breakfast, either. You'll be that much less hungry at lunch. And take a tip from Europe: Eat a light dinner. You may sleep better and wake up more refreshed.

In case you haven't noticed, you will continue to eat *"à la Français."* The French love their food and drink, yet they're slimmer on the whole than most Americans. Their rate of heart attacks is only one-third that of the United States. They're doing something right. Now, so are you.

A Few Final Tips
For the Maintenance Program

Watch What You Drink

Now that you're no longer on a diet, you'll probably want to go out with friends and to parties. Why refuse an invitation? But watch out: Two cocktails plus three glasses of wine provide significantly more calories than you're allowed on any weight-maintenance plan. See Table 4 on page 47 for the caloric content of some popular drinks —you may be surprised. However, if you have yielded to temptation, don't panic. Make up for your excesses the next day with a dinner from Stage Two of the Weight Loss Program. And enjoy yourself when you do it: Pick something from the Chef's Menu!

At the Office

Let's say you've yielded to a little temptation by nibbling on some gift chocolates with your colleagues. Make up for it in the evening. Select something from Stage One of the Preparation Program.

Actually, you're better off if you kick the nibbling habit for good. These types of foods usually supply your body with nothing more than sugar and fat. They contain none of the nutrients your body needs, and eating them regularly can lead to an unbalanced diet.

It's Your Child's or Husband's or Your Birthday

Anything goes! Go ahead and splurge. But make up for it the next day by selecting something from Stage Two of the Weight Loss Program or Stage One of the Preparation Program (depending on how bad you were). There's no reason why you can't take control of your eating habits. Stop that perpetual gain-again-diet-again cycle.

Eat More, Yes, But. . . .

Avoid eating very high-calorie foods at the same meal. It doesn't make sense to eat at one time:

a cocktail
an appetizer
a fatty dish

a high-fat cheese
a creamy dish
bread, and
wine

If you've eaten one fatty food, don't drink too much, and have fruit for dessert. Use your own good judgment.

At Home

Use the Chef's Menu as often as possible. There is a wide range to choose from, from soup to desserts—eighty-three delicious, original dishes. Most of these recipes are low in calories, even though their gourmet quotients are typically French. Try to incorporate these meals into your normal weekly menus, to bring back the joy of eating to yourself, your family, and your guests.

Even if you use the recipes only once in a while, keep the good eating habits outlined in Chapter 4. Don't use too much fat or salt. Follow the cooking and preparation guidelines in that chapter.

More than anything, enjoy yourself and enjoy your food. You now look better and feel healthier, so it shouldn't be hard.

The Maintenance Program: Stage Two

Summary for Easy Reference

At this stage of the diet, you should eat certain basic foods each day. These are listed in the summary that follows.

Refer to the exchange tables on page 185 to find out which foods are the exact equivalents of the ones listed. If you do make a substitution, be sure to use the exact quantities in the tables. For example, 1 cup of plain low-fat yogurt is equal to 1⅓ cups of skim milk. You could have either and adhere to the diet. However, if you drink 2 cups of skim milk in place of 1 cup of yogurt, you'd be consuming too many calories.

You might want to photocopy this summary page to have it with you when you're away from home, so you'll never doubt how much and what to eat.

The Maintenance Program: Stage Two

Summary Plan

BREAKFAST

3 slices plain bread (any type) with 2 pats butter or margarine; or
1 cup any cereal with ½ cup low fat milk; or 1 English muffin
with 1 pat butter or margarine

¾ cup plain low-fat yogurt or ¾ cup low-fat cottage cheese

1 tbs sugar, jelly, jam, or marmalade (can be used with yogurt,
cottage cheese, cereal, fruit, or beverage)

½ cup fruit juice or 1 piece fruit (can be saved for dessert at lunch
or dinner)

beverage

LUNCH

medium mixed or green salad with 1 tbs oil or regular salad dressing

1 low-calorie prepared meal or:

    1 cup cooked vegetables (boiled or steamed) or 2 cups raw
vegetables with 1 pat butter or margarine

4 oz lean meat or fish (cooked without oil or fat—baked, broiled,
steamed, or grilled only)

1 slice or 1 oz cheese with 1 slice plain bread (any type) or 4 plain
crackers

1 medium-size piece or ½ cup fruit

beverage

DINNER

medium mixed or green salad with 1 tbs oil or regular salad dressing

4 oz lean meat or fish (cooked without oil or fat—baked, broiled,
steamed, or grilled only)

3 medium potatoes or starchy foods (see exchange tables) with 1 pat
butter or margarine or 1 tbs sour cream

½ cup plain low-fat yogurt or ½ cup plain low-fat cottage cheese

beverage

For Men

At this calorie level, men no longer need to raise the amount of protein. Therefore, a husband and wife can now follow the same plan.

The Maintenance Program: Stage Two

The Standard Diet

The following menu plan is for one week of the 1,800-calorie Standard Diet. All the meals are simple to find and prepare but very satisfying. If you are going to follow this diet for two weeks or more, just repeat the week, and use the exchange tables to vary your meals. If you want to follow the Chef's Menu, use the menus for Stage One, and add food according to the guidelines included in this chapter.

DAY ONE

BREAKFAST
3 slices plain bread (any type)
  with 2 pats butter or
  margarine and 1 tbs jam,
  jelly, or marmalade
¾ cup plain low-fat yogurt with
  1 piece chopped fruit
beverage

LUNCH
medium green salad with 1 tbs
  oil or regular salad dressing
1 slice pizza (regular crust)
1 piece fruit
beverage

DINNER
medium mixed salad with 1 tbs
  oil or regular salad dressing
4 oz broiled lean meat
1 cup cooked corn, winter
  squash, or peas
1 slice plain bread (any type) or
  4 plain crackers
1 cup plain low-fat yogurt with
  1 piece chopped fruit
beverage

DAY TWO

BREAKFAST
1 cup any cereal with ½ cup
low-fat milk and 1 tbs sugar
¾ cup low-fat cottage cheese
with 1 piece chopped fruit
½ cup orange juice
beverage

LUNCH
medium green salad with 1 tbs
oil or regular salad dressing
3–4 oz individual can of water-
packed tuna or salmon
2 slices plain bread (any type) or
8 plain crackers
1 piece fruit
beverage

DINNER
medium bowl vegetable soup
4 oz roasted chicken or turkey
1 cup cooked mixed vegetables,
carrots, or peas with 1 pat
butter or margarine
1 slice or 1 oz low-fat cheese
1 slice plain bread (any type) or
4 plain crackers
½ cup plain low-fat yogurt
1 apple
beverage: 2 glasses of wine or 2
6-oz glasses of soda or fruit
juice

DAY THREE

BREAKFAST
¾ cup plain low-fat yogurt with
1 piece chopped fruit
1 cup orange juice
beverage

LUNCH
small mixed salad with 1 tbs oil
or regular salad dressing
4 oz cold chicken or chicken
breast
1 cup cooked broccoli, Brussels
sprouts, or spinach
1 slice or 1 oz cheese with
4 plain crackers
1 cup mixed fruit salad
beverage

DINNER
medium green salad with 2 tbs
   oil or regular salad dressing
4 oz broiled or baked fish
1 baked potato with 1 tbs sour
   cream or 1 pat butter or
   margarine
¾ cup low-fat cottage cheese
   with 1 piece chopped fruit
beverage

DAY FOUR

BREAKFAST
1 cup any cereal with ½ cup
   low-fat milk and 1 tbs sugar
½ cup plain low-fat yogurt
½ cup grapefruit juice
beverage

LUNCH
large chef's salad (2 oz turkey,
   2 oz ham, 2 oz cheese,
   lettuce, 1 medium tomato)
   with 1 tbs oil or regular salad
   dressing
1 piece fruit
beverage

DINNER
medium tomato salad with 1 tbs
   oil or regular salad dressing
4 oz trout, sole, or snapper
1 cup cooked rice with 1 pat
   butter or margarine
½ cup plain low-fat yogurt
beverage: 2 glasses of wine or 2
   6-oz glasses of soda or fruit
   juice

DAY FIVE

BREAKFAST
1 English muffin with 1 pat
   butter or margarine
¾ cup low-fat cottage cheese
   with 1 piece chopped fruit
½ cup orange juice
beverage

LUNCH
large mixed salad with 1 tbs oil
   or regular salad dressing
4 oz broiled beef, chicken, or
   shrimp
1 slice or 1 oz cheese with
   4 plain crackers
1 piece fruit
beverage

DINNER
medium green salad with 1 tbs
   oil or regular salad dressing
1 low-calorie frozen prepared
   meal or 1 cup cooked mixed
   vegetables and 4 oz lean fish
1 slice plain bread (any type) or
   4 plain crackers
1 cup ice cream
beverage

DAY SIX

BREAKFAST
1 cup any cereal with ½ cup
   low-fat milk and 1 tbs sugar
¾ cup plain low-fat yogurt
½ cup orange juice
beverage

LUNCH
medium green salad with 1 tbs
   oil or regular salad dressing
4 oz lean hamburger with 1 slice
   or 1 oz cheese
1 hamburger bun
small portion of French fries
¾ plain low-fat yogurt with
   1 piece chopped fruit
beverage

DINNER
medium mixed salad with 1 tbs
    oil or regular salad dressing
4 oz lean veal
1 cup cooked cabbage or
    Brussels sprouts with 1 pat
    butter or margarine
1 slice or 1 oz cheese with
    4 crackers
1 piece fruit
beverage

DAY SEVEN

BREAKFAST
3 slices plain bread (any type)
    with 2 pats butter or
    margarine and 1 tbs jam,
    jelly, or marmalade
¾ cup plain low-fat yogurt
½ cup orange juice
beverage

LUNCH
large mixed salad with 1 tbs oil
    or regular salad dressing
1 leg or 4 oz cold roast chicken
1½ cups yellow corn with 1 pat
    butter or margarine
beverage

DINNER
medium bowl vegetable soup
4 oz broiled fish (any kind)
1 cup cooked spinach or
    broccoli with 1 pat butter or
    margarine
½ cup plain low-fat yogurt with
    1 piece chopped fruit
beverage: 1 6-oz glass of beer or
    1 6-oz glass of fruit juice or
    soda

The Maintenance Program: Stage Three

Summary for Easy Reference

At this, the highest stage of the Maintenance Program, you should eat certain basic foods each day. These are listed below.

Refer to the exchange tables on page 185 to find out which foods are the exact equivalents of the ones listed. If you do make a substitution, use the exact quantities in the tables. For example, 1 cup of plain low-fat yogurt is equal to 1⅓ cups of skim milk. You could have either and adhere to the diet. However, if you drink 2 cups of skim milk in place of 1 cup of yogurt, you'd be taking in too many calories.

You might want to photocopy this summary page to have it with you when you're away from home, so you'll never be in doubt about how much and what to eat.

The Maintenance Program: Stage Three

Summary Plan

BREAKFAST

3 slices plain bread (any type) with 2 pats butter or margarine; or 1 cup any cereal with ½ cup low-fat milk; or 1 English muffin with 1 pat butter or margarine

¾ cup plain low-fat yogurt or ¾ cup low-fat cottage cheese

1 tbs sugar or 1 tbs jelly, jam, or marmalade (can be used with yogurt, cottage cheese, cereal, fruit, or beverage)

½ cup fruit juice or 1 piece fruit (can be saved for lunch or dinner)

beverage

LUNCH

medium mixed or green salad with 1 tbs oil or regular salad dressing

1 low-calorie prepared frozen meal or:

    1 cup cooked vegetables (boiled or steamed) or 2 cups raw vegetables with 1 pat butter or margarine

4 oz lean meat or fish (cooked without oil or fat—baked, broiled,
  steamed, or grilled only)
1 slice or 1 oz cheese with 1 slice plain bread (any type) or 4 plain
  crackers
1 medium-size piece or ½ cup fruit
beverage

DINNER

medium mixed or green salad with 2 tbs oil or regular salad dressing
4 oz lean meat or fish (cooked without oil or fat—baked, broiled,
  steamed, or grilled only)
3 medium potatoes or starchy foods (see exchange tables) with 1 pat
  butter or margarine
¾ cup plain low-fat yogurt with 1 piece chopped fruit, or ¾ cup
  low-fat cottage cheese with 1 piece chopped fruit, or ½ cup ice
  cream
beverage

For Men

At this calorie level, men no longer need to raise the amount of
protein. Therefore, a husband and wife can now follow the same
plan.

PART SIX

❦

Accompaniments,
Exercise
and
Clarification

CHAPTER 12

The Exercise Plan

*Y*ou may need an extra "push" while dieting, a boost of energy to perk you up and make you feel great. In addition, you'll want that new, leaner body to become firm and tight, shown off to its best advantage. You can get all these things and more through exercise. Exercise will tone up your body, inside and out. It can make you feel and be healthier than ever before. And it's not as painful or difficult as some people make it out to be—that is, not if you follow the right program.

As an essential companion to the diet, we offer you our exercise plan. It works perfectly with the program. Do these workouts at least five days a week while dieting (you can take weekends off) and at least three days a week while on the Maintenance Program and beyond. It's a good idea to schedule the exercises for the same time of the day, so they become a ritual. Once you start working out regularly, you will probably find that you miss the invigoration and relaxation it brings when you skip a session. For this reason, many people choose to exercise every day of the week for at least twenty minutes.

We also would like to point out, right at the start, that no one should undertake any program of regular exercise without first consulting a physician. As healthy as working out is, an overly strenuous program can be dangerous for people with certain conditions, such as heart disease. Tell your physician about your routine and let him or her decide if it's right for you.

While it's hard to lose weight through exercise alone (see Chapter 2), it's hard to look and feel great through dieting alone. The two work hand in hand, and exercise actually helps the process of dieting.

Let us explain. Through regular workouts, the body burns off more fat by increasing its metabolic rate. For example, let's say you hop on the exercise bicycle and ride for thirty minutes each morning. Not only will your body work off a certain number of calories, but it will also continue to use more than normal throughout the morning. Once it's warmed up, it becomes like a motor that keeps humming and burning fuel.

In addition to burning off more fat, exercise also increases your energy level, keeps your heart healthy, raises HDL (the good cholesterol), and improves circulation. Your skin, hair, eyes, and body will all look their best. Isn't a better appearance and better health the main reasons why you're dieting?

The Components of a Good Workout

There are three parts to this program:

1. aerobic exercise that burns off calories;
2. strengthening exercises that improve muscle tone; and
3. flexibility exercises that increase the range of motion in your joints.

Some strengthening and flexibility are important to protect you from injury while exercising and must be included in every workout program. If you don't loosen your limbs first, you might pull or tear something during the aerobics, such as jogging. The aerobic section of the plan is the most important for weight loss.

You should understand that, in order to get the most out of the program, everyone must work at their own pace. Just because your best friend (who has been going to a gym for two years) can do thirty repetitions of every exercise with ease doesn't mean that you (who haven't worked out for ten years) can do the same. It's dangerous, and it's damaging to your psyche. If you try to do too much at first, your limbs will ache, you'll feel miserable, and chances are you'll stop exercising. Work it up slowly and surely, and your body will respond beautifully. Remember, this program is for your enjoyment; you can tailor our suggestions to your own pace and your own favorite exercises. We've given you a wide range of options.

Most of All, Do It!

Working out has a few basic requirements:

1. you have to donate a little chunk of time each day;
2. you have to change clothes;
3. you have to sweat; and
4. you have to breathe properly.

Practice inhaling and exhaling deeply. Lie on your back facing a mirror and breathe. See if you can push down toward your lower spine and get your tummy to raise and lower with each breath. If your chest is the only thing that's moving, your breaths are too shallow. You'll feel much better with deep breathing. Try this simple exercise: Inhale for four slow counts, raising your tummy, hold it there for eight counts, then slowly exhale for four counts. Do this four times. You'll probably feel an immediate sense of relaxation and stimulation.

Take a look at these "get-going" tips every now and then. You may want to add to them when you discover some of your own:

• Any exercise is better than no exercise. If you can't complete your workout in the morning because a new client (or admirer) is meeting you for breakfast, then finish it in the evening.

• Workout with a friend; you'll keep each other going. If it's the new (or old) admirer, it can become a sensuous experience.

• Keep in mind that you'll always feel better after a workout. Remember how good you felt the last time?

• If you are riding a stationary bicycle, watch a television program, read a book or magazine, or listen to some inspiring music.

• Buy a new workout outfit or new exercise shoes.

• For running or fast walking by yourself, pick a scenic spot or listen to music with headphones.

• Find the most "excuse-less" time of day to exercise, and stick to it. Don't start your workout in the middle of the afternoon when chores, phone calls, or business demands can distract you.

• Unless you are devoted to one type of exercise, such as tennis, vary your program as much as possible to avoid boredom.

Your Target Heart Rate

You'll need to learn how to regulate the intensity at which you're exercising. This enables you to know if you're overworking or not going at it hard enough. By taking your pulse during your workouts, you'll find out when you've reached your target heart rate (THR)— the right intensity to burn off calories.

To calculate your THR, take the number 220 and subtract your age. This will give you the estimated maximum heart rate (MHR). Now, multiply the MHR by 70 percent to get the THR. For example, let's say you're thirty years old:

$$\begin{array}{cc} 220 & 190 \\ \underline{-\ 30} & \underline{\times .70} \\ 190\ \text{MHR} & 133\ \text{THR} \end{array}$$

Your THR is 133 beats per minute. THRs can vary anywhere from 60 percent to 85 percent of your MHR. For this program, beginners start at the lower end of the range. However, if you are in very good physical condition, you can workout at 80–85 percent of your MHR. Let's follow this rule:

1. Beginners work out at 60–65 percent of MHR;
2. Intermediates work out at 70–75 percent; and
3. Advanced work out at 80–85 percent.

As your fitness level increases, you should increase your THR accordingly.

Take your pulse in the following way: Place your right index and third fingers gently on the carotid artery in your neck (on the side) or on the radial artery of your wrist (inside edges), and feel for your pulse. When you find it, count the beats for ten seconds (using a stopwatch or second hand of your wristwatch). Multiply the figure you get by six. Practice a few times before exercising.

Take your pulse before you begin your workout, then repeat every ten minutes. You should reach your THR somewhere toward the middle of the routine. For maximum benefit, don't go above or below it. If you find that it's going too high, slow down and cool off. Before proceeding to the next exercise, your pulse should be below 120 (a count of twenty for ten seconds).

During the preparation stage of the Paris Diet, the exercise program will teach you how to strengthen and tone up your body and to develop a workout regimen. The weight-loss stage will include only toning exercises since you shouldn't be exercising too strenuously while on very low-calorie diets. During the Adjustment and Maintenance Programs, the focus will be on gradually building up your muscular strength and cardiovascular endurance. The stronger you are, the harder your body can work to burn off calories. Do not exercise to exhaustion during any stage; instead, work at a consistent, but comfortable intensity.

Warm-Up and Cool-Down Exercises for All Stages: Preparation Through Maintenance

These exercises start and end each workout. They will loosen and strengthen your body for the more intense parts of the program. Do them in the order that they are listed here.

The basic warm-ups and cool-downs should last anywhere from three to eight minutes. Keep your pulse rate at no more than 60–75 percent of the MHR.

Moving March

Function (what it does): Gets blood flowing to the extremities.

Movement (how to do it): Walk in place. Lift knees high toward chest. Push legs off the floor with pointed toes. Bend elbows and pump arms back and forth like a speed skater.

Alignment (correct position of your body): Abdominal (stomach) muscles are tight. Upper body is slightly forward. Lift legs from back of thighs and hips. Don't lock your knees when straightening them back down on the floor.

Static Stretch

Function: Stretches back of calf and shin.

Movement: Stand 1½ to 2 feet from wall, facing it. Step forward with right leg and bend right knee. Lean forward with upper body and place hands on wall at shoulder level. Hold stretch for thirty seconds. Repeat with left leg.

Alignment: Keep back leg straight, with heel on floor. Keep abdominals tight and press hip bones forward. Tilt pelvis forward and keep back heel on floor.

Quad Stretch
Function: To strengthen muscles in top of thigh.
Movement: Standing upright, place hand on wall for support. Bend right knee and grasp right ankle with right hand, pulling foot to hip behind you. Hold foot for thirty seconds while stretching out the top of your thigh. Repeat on left side.
Alignment: Keep abdominals tight and do not allow back to arch.

Spinal-Abdominal Warm Up
Function: To warm up spine and stomach muscles.
Movement: Standing upright, inhale, then exhale. Tilt pelvis forward by tightening abdominal muscles (as if you were punched in the stomach). Allow arms to stretch forward and drop head. Hold for five seconds, then release.
Alignment: Stand with feet apart about shoulder width. Bend knees slightly. Do not tighten lower back muscles. Imagine tightening the abdominals and stretching out the lower back. Hollow out your middle. Begin the movement with your abdominals.

Workout For Weight Loss Program Only

Since the Preparation, Adjustment, and Maintenance Programs of the workout are the same and take longer, we will start with the exercises for the Weight Loss Program. Do this while following the Weight Loss Program. DO NOT DO ANY AEROBIC EXERCISE DURING THE WEIGHT LOSS PROGRAM. Do only these workouts. They will keep your body strong, well-shaped, and toned but will not tax it too much. They will also give you an energy boost when you need it most.

Start with the basic warm-ups just described. Then, begin these workouts on the floor. Do them in order, again keeping your THR at the low end.

Lower Back Stretch I

Function: To stretch abdominals and lower back.

Movement: Lie on the floor on your back. Bring right knee into chest. Hug arms around right knee. Slide left leg straight out onto floor. Hold six seconds. Bring nose to right knee. Hold six seconds. Inhale, exhale, then bring both knees into chest. Inhale, exhale, Hold six seconds. Repeat with left knee.

Alignment: Keep abdominals tight and back pressed to floor. Feel stretch from top of head to toes.

Cat Stretch I

Function: To strengthen and stretch lower back.

Movement: Roll over onto hands and knees, weight evenly distributed. Tighten abdominals and round back like a cat. Pull belly button up toward lower back. Hold ten seconds. Keeping abdominals tight, straighten out spine. Repeat five times.

Alignment: Make movements smooth and even, always using abdominals.

Cat Stretch II

Function: To strengthen abdominals.

Movement: Start in same position as Cat Stretch I. Roll down to forearms so you're in slanted position, hips pointed behind you. Tighten abdominal muscles. Pull belly button up toward spine. Hold ten seconds, release. Exhale as you pull up; inhale as you release. Repeat ten times.

Alignment: Same as Cat Stretch I.

Abdominal Curl-Ups

Function: To strengthen lower abdominal muscles.

Movement: Roll onto back. Bend knees. Leave feet on floor, directly under knees. Place hands behind head with elbows opened out to sides. Inhale and fill tummy with air; exhale and tighten abdominal muscles while slowly lifting upper body off floor to the count of two. Keeping abdominals tight, slowly lower upper body to floor, not allowing elbows to touch. Repeat six times, gradually working up at your own pace to thirty repetitions.

Alignment: Make sure abdominals stay tight during entire exercise. Chest and face are always lifted toward ceiling. Do not try to curl toward your knees, like a traditional sit-up. Always lift up toward ceiling. Imagine "shaping" your stomach muscles to the way you want them to look. Always imagine "scooping" or "hollowing out" your abdominals. Never push them out when lifting. Work abdominal muscles below the belly button.

Advanced Abdominals

Function: To further strengthen lower abdominal muscles.

Movement: Start in same position as Abdominal Curl-Ups. Exhale and tighten lower abdominals and lift half way up; hold for one count. Lift higher by tightening lower abdominals again; hold for one count. Lower for two counts, keeping lower abdominal muscles tight. Repeat ten times; increase repetitions by five as you progress to a maximum of thirty.

Alignment: See Abdominal Curl-Ups.

Oblique Curl-Ups

Function: To strengthen oblique muscles (under rib cage and above hip bone).

Movement: Start in same position as Abdominal Curl-Ups. Cross right ankle over left knee. Stretch right arm straight out to side with palm down on floor at shoulder level; left hand is cupped behind head. Tighten oblique muscles (under right rib cage and above right hip bone); hold for one count. Bring left elbow across to right knee and lower. When down, keep back pressed against floor. Repeat on left side. For first five days of doing exercise, repeat five times; for second five days and beyond, repeat ten times.

Alignment: See Abdominal Curl-Ups.

Lower Back Stretch II

Function: To stretch out abdominals and relax lower back.

Movement: Repeat the Lower Back Stretch I.

Thigh Strengthener

Function: To strengthen outer thigh.

Movement: Lie on right side, right arm stretched out above head on floor, head resting on arm. Fold both knees into chest to make a right angle in front of body, knees pointed away from belly button. Lean body forward and tighten outside of left thigh to lift leg two to three inches off floor. Lift on one count, hold one count, lower for one count. Repeat with right leg, lying on left side. Repeat five times each side, increasing at your own pace to fifteen repetitions.

Alignment: Keep legs parallel, abdominals tight, toes pointed.

Thigh-Hip Stretch

Function: To stretch outer thigh and hip.

Movement: Sit cross-legged on floor, right leg in front, both hips on floor. Lean forward with upper body, placing hands on floor. Twist upper body to left diagonally so that you're stretching over left knee. Slide right hand forward and press right hip into floor. Hold thirty seconds, then repeat on left side.

Alignment: Make sure hips are pressed into floor. Do not try to twist upper body all the way to the side; twist only to diagonal position.

Gluteal/Hamstring Strengthener

Function: To strengthen gluteals (buttocks) and hamstrings (back of thigh).

Movement: Lie face down, elbows bent out to sides. Hands are folded under chin with palms down. Point legs straight out on floor. Tighten buttocks, press hip bones into floor, and contract right buttocks to slowly lift right leg two inches off floor. Lower, repeat with left buttocks and leg. Begin with five repetitions, work up at your own pace to fifteen.

Alignment: Keep front of hip and thigh on floor. Don't use lower back. Point toes. If lower back tightens, stop and bring knees into chest for count of twenty to relax.

Inner Thigh Strengthener

Function: To strengthen and tighten inner thigh.

Movement: Lie on right side, right arm stretched above head on

floor, head resting on arm. Bend left leg and rest on floor in front
of right leg. Keep right leg straight, tighten inner thigh and lift
right leg four to five inches off floor. Hold one count, lower.
Repeat on left side. Start with five times, build up to fifteen.
Alignment: Keep inner thighs facing ceiling, lifted leg straight.

Inner Thigh and Ham Stretch
Function: To stretch inner and back of thigh.
Movement: Sit on floor in straddle position (legs open to sides). Bend
and slide left leg in so foot touches inner thigh. Lean upper body
forward and hold for fifteen counts. Relax. Slide right leg directly
in front of you. Keep left leg in place. Lean forward to stretch out
back of right leg. Hold for fifteen counts. Relax. Repeat on left
side.
Alignment: Keep hips on floor, knees pointed toward ceiling. Flex
foot of straight leg.

Pectoral Strengthener
Function: To strengthen pectoral (front of shoulder) muscles.
Movement: Sit cross-legged. Open arms straight out to sides at shoulder level. Bend elbows to make right angles with both arms, fingers
pointed toward ceiling. Tighten front of shoulders and bring elbows together in front of you. Hold one count, then open back
out. Repeat ten times.
Alignment: Keep abdominals tight. Keep elbows lifted to shoulder
level at all times. Use muscle in front of shoulder to open arms
back out.

Workout for Preparation, Adjustment and Maintenance Programs

These exercises can be done during all but the Weight Loss Program.
At your own pace, gradually build up your time and intensity. Remember to check with your doctor before beginning any exercise
progam.
Plan to spend at least five to fifteen minutes at least three times a

week on these workouts; gradually build it up at your own pace. Thirty minutes maximum is best for the Preparation and Adjustment Programs; build up to an hour if you can by the Maintenance Program.

1. For all stages, start with the basic warm-ups.
2. Follow with an aerobic segment. We have included our own special walk and walk/jog program that many people find easy to do. However, if you want to substitute your own favorite exercise, go right ahead. Here are some suggestions for good aerobic workouts:

- walking: everyone starts at fifteen minutes, gradually working up to an hour.
- jogging: beginners start at five minutes, working up to thirty; intermediate-advanced start at fifteen minutes, work up to a full hour.
- combo walk/jog: see program that follows.
- bicycle (stationary or outdoor): beginners start with eight minutes, working up to forty; advanced start with fifteen minutes, working up to sixty.
- swimming: beginners start at ten minutes, working up to forty-five; advanced start at fifteen minutes, working up to sixty.
- jogging in pool (good for people with injuries, arthritis): beginners start at five minutes, working up to twenty-five; advanced start with fifteen minutes, working up to forty.
- treadmill (walking indoors): everyone starts at fifteen minutes, working up to sixty.
- cross-country ski machine: beginners start at eight minutes, working up to thirty; advanced start at fifteen minutes, working up to one hour.
- aerobics classes (low impact or combo high/low impact for advanced): beginners start with sixty-minute beginners' classes with twenty-minute aerobic segment (march or walk in place when tired); advanced begin with sixty-minute class with twenty-minute intermediate-level aerobic segment (advanced should work up to ninety-minute advanced classes with forty-five to sixty-minute aerobic segment).

- rowing (machine or outdoors): beginners start with ten minutes, working up to thirty; advanced start at twenty minutes,
working up to forty-five.

Always remember to do the Basic Warm-Up prior to workout. Use
the Static Stretches to cool down.

3. Take your pulse before the warm-up and every ten minutes
following, plus after the cool-down. Don't go above your THR, and
don't start another exercise after cool-down until your pulse rate has
reached 120 or lower. Beginners should keep their workout intensity
at 60–75 percent of the MHR; advanced exercisers can work at 70–
85 percent.

4. Begin the aerobic segment gradually. Slowly work up the time
and intensity. Neither Rome nor Paris was built in a day! Always
make sure you're not gasping for air but are able to talk while
working out.

5. Work out at a consistent, steady pace. Exercising at high intensity and then stopping is not the way to burn off fat.

The Walk Program

Beginners: Keep heart rate at low end of THR (60–75 percent of
MHR).
Intermediate-Advanced: Keep heart rate at 70–85 percent of MHR.

Begin walking slowly, gradually increasing your speed to reach
your THR. Allow your arms to swing freely; keep abdominals tight
and trunk erect, with pelvis tipped slightly forward. Keep feet point-
ing forward and roll heel, ball, toe as you walk. Keep rib cage relaxed
and breathe from below your diaphram (around your belly button).
Walk through relaxing places (like parks, suburbs) and/or use headphones for music.

Schedule for Walk Program

Keep a notebook to record how long and how often you walk, and
your heart rate range. Try to walk every day. Recent studies have
shown that people who walk for just a half hour a day can lose fifteen

to twenty pounds in a year without cutting out one single calorie. They also have great legs!

DAY	DURATION (MINUTES)
1	15
2	20
3	20
4	25
5	25
6	30
7	30
8	30
9	30
10	35
11	35
12	40
13	40
14	45
15	45
16	45
17	45
18	45
19	50
20	50
21	55
22 and beyond	60

If you want to simplify the walk program, use the following schedule:

WEEK ONE: 20–30 minutes
WEEK TWO: 30–40 minutes
WEEK THREE: 40–50 minutes
WEEK FOUR: 50–60 minutes

After week four, continue walking for sixty minutes at a brisk pace.

Walk/Jog Program (Maintenance Program Only)

If you want to further build your physical strength and endurance, begin this program after completing week three of the walk program, instead of going on to week four and beyond of straight walking. Start each walk/jog session with the basic warm-ups. Cool down and end each session with the Static Stretches from the Basic Warm-Up.

For each phase of this workout, note how you feel. Do not proceed to the next phase if you are uncomfortable. Exercise should be a self-loving, sensuous experience, not torture. You may want to work on each phase for several days or even weeks. Keep your pulse at the low end of the THR, but move continuously without making uneven stops and starts. Take your pulse constantly to check your workout intensity, and use a brisk walk to lower your heart rate when necessary. Use a pumping action with your arms to maintain the heart rate when doing a brisk walk, and always keep your chest lifted.

Do the walk/jog every other day. Do brisk walking for twenty minutes and the workouts for the Weight Loss Program on alternate days. Or if you don't want to do this program, just stick to the walking plan.

Remember, don't follow this or any other exercise program before you have checked with your doctor.

Schedule for Walk/Jog

PHASE 1
Total Workout Time: 25 minutes
Brisk Walk: 10 minutes
Take your pulse, if okay, work into a
Slow Jog: 5 minutes, then cool down with a
Brisk Walk: 10 minutes, gradually slowing down at end

PHASE 2
Total Workout Time: 30 minutes
Walk: 5 minutes
Jog: 5 minutes
Take pulse
Walk: 5 minutes

Jog: 5 minutes
Take pulse
Walk: 10 minutes, gradually slowing down at end

PHASE 3
Total Workout Time: 30–35 minutes
Walk: 5 minutes
Jog: 10–15 minutes
Check pulse and walk when necessary
Walk: 15 minutes, very briskly, gradually slowing down at end

PHASE 4
Total Workout Time: 30 minutes
Walk: 5 minutes
Jog: 20 minutes
Take pulse
Walk: 5 minutes, very briskly, gradually slowing down at end

PHASE 5
Total Workout Time: 35–40 minutes
Walk: 5 minutes
Jog: 25–30 minutes
Walk: 5 minutes, very briskly, gradually slowing down at end

For these phases, cool down by walking at a normal pace. Check to see that your pulse is below 120 beats per minute, then finish off with the Static Stretches. Remember, do not proceed to the next phase until you are comfortable with the one you're doing.

Try all or some of these workouts while you're on the Paris Diet and afterward. Remember that weight loss alone is not enough. Careful, proper exercise can make that slimmer body look ten years younger, be healthier and stronger, and feel wonderful.

CHAPTER 13

Answers to Your Questions About the Paris Diet

*A*lthough it has many programs, the Paris Diet is easy to follow and easier to enjoy. However, some people still have questions about how it works, especially under certain conditions. Here are all the answers you'll need to make the program work to your best advantage.

Can I stay on the Weight Loss Program for longer than four weeks?

Yes. There's no harm in remaining at Stage One of the Weight Loss Program for an extra week because the diet is well balanced and varied, and you'll be taking the vitamins and minerals your body needs in a daily supplement. But there's no point in staying on this stage if you only have a few more pounds (five to ten) to shed. Exercise and sensible eating will take care of that.

If you have over fifteen pounds more to lose, stay on Stage One for another week, then move to Stage Two for ten to fourteen days. But remember that the rest of the program must be followed exactly; in other words, don't cut weeks off other stages because you've added a week to the Weight Loss Program. The Adjustment and Maintenance Programs are just as important to the overall plan.

What if I don't lose weight the first time around?

There's practically no reason why you shouldn't be able to lose significant amounts of weight on the Paris Diet. It's unusual but it might occur if you started taking certain drugs, which may cause weight gain. Ask your doctor if you're taking any medications that can have this effect.

If you're taking such drugs, you may not lose weight, but on the other hand, you won't gain weight either. So the diet is still of benefit. These types of medical treatments are usually temporary, and there's no reason not to lose weight once you stop taking the drugs.

If you go on the diet at the same time you quit smoking, you also may not lose any weight, but in this case the object of the program would be to stop you from gaining. When smokers quit, they can gain from eight to thirty pounds.

Still having a problem? Then you aren't following the diet. Maybe you're sneaking a snack every now and then, or drinking "just a shot" of alcohol. This diet is precisely calculated and must be followed as it is written. Do not miss any meals, and do not add anything to the meals. One little apple may not seem like much, but it can upset the whole cart.

You may have skipped the Preparation Program and gone right to the Weight Loss Program. If you've been dieting all your life, skipping these stages will defeat the purpose of the program. You have to eat more at first and get your metabolism back to normal before you can eat less and lose significant amounts of weight.

How much will I lose on this program?

If you're twenty to thirty pounds overweight, the Paris Diet will help you lose it and slim down once and for all. You'll never have to diet again, and you'll probably be eating more than you did before.

If you're more than thirty pounds over your ideal weight, you might have to go through the program twice. However, it's essential that you stay on the Maintenance Program for at least one month before starting the plan over again.

I eat more than 1,800 calories a day. Should I start on the
Preparation Program?

No. People who are significantly overweight, large, or eat over 1,400 calories a day (most men fall into this category) don't have to follow the Preparation Program. The preparatory phase is intended for light eaters or for those who dieted less than two months previous to this. Heavier eaters usually start with the Weight Loss Program.

On the other hand, people who are heavy eaters but have less than twenty pounds to lose can skip the Weight Loss Program. The

Adjustment and Maintenance Programs will help them shed weight. These people should follow the Adjustment Program for a month, go on to the Maintenance Program, starting with Stage One for two weeks, then follow with Stages Two and Three for a month.

I've never been on a diet before. How should I follow the program?

If you've never been on a diet before or were on a diet over two months ago, start with the Weight Loss Program; stay at Stage One for two weeks, then move to Stage Two for two more weeks. Then go to Stage One of the Adjustment Program for another two weeks —you may continue to lose weight on this plan, especially if you consumed a lot of calories before and have never been on a diet.

Next, move up to Stage Two of the Adjustment Program. The longer you stay on this stage, the greater your chances of keeping the weight off for good; one full month would be best. Likewise, when you move on to the Maintenance Program, stay on Stages One and Two for one month each. Remember, once you're up to Stage Two of the Adjustment Program, you'll be eating normally, not sticking to a terribly limited diet. You are just increasing your food intake naturally and gradually—without gaining weight the way you used to do. The diet works very well even if you stay on the stages of the Adjustment Program for two weeks each. Our experience has shown, however, that people with the highest permanent weight loss are those who stayed on them for the whole month.

I don't eat much at all and yet can't seem to lose any weight. My highest food intake is around 1,400 calories and often drops to as low as 1,000 calories a day. My last diet was a month ago and I only lost three quarters of a pound! Will this program work for me? What should I do?

The Preparation Program of the Paris Diet has been designed especially for you. Within a month of starting it—two weeks at Stage One and two weeks at Stage Two—your body will gradually learn to take in more without putting on a single ounce. There's even a good chance you'll lose two to six pounds since the diet is varied and rich in protein. After the first month, follow the steps of the rest of the program as follows:

1. The Weight Loss Program: Stage One for two weeks;
2. The Weight Loss Program: Stage Two for two weeks;
3. The Adjustment Program: Stage One for two weeks;
4. The Adjustment Program: Stage Two for two to four weeks;
5. The Maintenance Program: Stage One for two to four weeks;
6. The Maintenance Program: Stage Two for two to four weeks.

In a minimum of six weeks, you can lose a great deal of weight and train your body to eat happily without ever gaining a pound. And you'll never have to diet again! That's certainly worth this relatively slight investment of time.

I'm a very heavy eater. Will I have to stay on the diet longer?

Because you do eat a lot, you'll lose weight more easily and quickly than most people. If you normally consume more than 3,000 calories a day and need to lose only twenty pounds, simply start with Stage Two of the Adjustment Program, and then follow the three stages of the Maintenance Program for two weeks each.

If you eat between 2,500 and 3,000 calories per day, start with Stage One of the Adjustment Program for two weeks, then move to Stage Two; and finally the full three stages of the Maintenance Program for two weeks each to reach your desired weight.

If you eat between 2,000 and 2,500 calories per day, start with the Weight Loss Program, then go to the Adjustment and Maintenance Programs.

Finally, it all depends on how fast you want to lose those extra pounds. Actually, there's no reason why even a heavy eater (over 3,000 calories daily) can't start with the Weight Loss Program. The weight will just come off more quickly.

I have to attend a lot of business lunches and cocktail parties. Will I still be able to lose weight on the Paris Diet?

To tell you the truth, even though this diet is varied and delicious, to make it work requires some self-discipline and sustained effort. It's difficult to combine business lunches (all drinking is out!) with the Weight Loss Program. Cocktail parties are even trickier (all those drinks, all those starchy and fatty hors d'oeuvres). If you accept a couple of lunch dates during the Weight Loss Program, stick rigidly to the foods you're allowed and to the quantities and the methods of cooking. For example, you could have a broiled shish kebab, green bean side course, and a fruit salad without sugar for lunch. Upon request, most restaurants will give you a plain grilled fish, a salad with a few lemon wedges and no dressing, and plain fresh berries for dessert. If you don't have to eat out, try our sample meals for the office.

Things will get easier on the Adjustment and Maintenance Programs. Try to limit yourself to two business lunches and one cocktail party a week, unless you can stick to our food selections. Many business people become almost obese from "socializing."

I need to lose over forty pounds. How long will it take?

"Lose fifty pounds in a month!" "Get rid of all your unwanted fat in two weeks!" "Shed twenty pounds a week and eat anything you want!"

By now most people realize that such slogans are false. No one can tell you exactly how much weight you'll lose within a week or a month. Each person is unique, with his or her own metabolism. Age, sex, physical activity, and eating habits all figure into the amount of weight lost on any program.

A man who normally eats a lot will lose more weight than a woman who eats very little, even if they follow the same diet. (However, the Preparation Program of the Paris Diet makes it possible for very light eaters to lose as much as those whose food intake is normal or slightly above average.)

A woman who's just had a baby or who is entering menopause will lose slightly less weight than an ordinary thirty-year-old woman even if she eats the same number of calories. But that doesn't mean that she can't lose the weight she wants by following our program.

If you're forty pounds or more overweight, you'll have to go through the Weight Loss, Adjustment, and Maintenance Programs twice, with an interval of at least one month between each cycle. You're better off taking the time to permanently lose the weight than to risk following a crash diet and then gain back every pound once you resume your normal eating habits.

If I go off the diet and splurge just once, will it still work?

Yes, if you slip for one day; it won't work if you splurge for several days in a row. Then there's a good chance you'll stop losing altogether and may even put some pounds back on!

During the Weight Loss Program, we strongly advise against "cheating." You could stop losing weight and for reasons still unknown, not lose weight again even when you resume the plan. Don't take the risk. Wait until you're on the Maintenance Program to go on the occasional food binge. Even at that stage, compensate for each lapse on the same day or the day after by following a lower calorie plan for a day or two.

Only when your weight has become stable—after several weeks on Stages Two and Three of the Maintenance Program—can you from time to time indulge yourself and eat some favorite but fattening foods.

Can this diet be used to control weight during pregnancy?

Pregnant women need to eat more calories than nonpregnant women (the energy cost of pregnancy is about 80,000 extra calories). Therefore, it's not a good time to diet since eating too little might prevent your baby from growing at a normal rate.

However, your doctor may have two reasons to prescribe a low-calorie diet at this time: If you were already seriously overweight when you became pregnant; or if you've put on too much weight during the course of your pregnancy.

In these cases, you may have to diet, but it can't be just any program. It must be a well-balanced plan that offers proper nutrition for both mother and child. Strict low-calorie plans can endanger the child. It can cause a low birth weight and put a child at risk for both physical and mental handicaps.

There's no danger if you follow Stage One of the Maintenance Program, but only—and we repeat ONLY—under your doctor's supervision. We give this diet to overweight pregnant women at the Bichat Hospital.

Your doctor can prescribe any necessary vitamin and mineral supplements, as well as take frequent tests to see how the baby is progressing in terms of weight and size.

If you do follow this plan, during the last three months of pregnancy replace the 2 ounces of meat with 1 ounce of hard cheese to cover the baby's calcium needs.

I'm slightly overweight and my cholesterol level is too high. Is the Paris Diet okay for someone like me?

One reason your cholesterol may be too high is because you're overweight. In other words, if you lose weight on the Paris Diet, your blood cholesterol levels could fall by as much as 20 percent.

Your present way of eating may be too rich in cholesterol and saturated fats and too poor in the right sorts of fats—monounsaturated and polyunsaturated fatty acids. This may increase the risk of hypercholesterolemia and coronary artery disease, especially in people who have a predisposition to such conditions.

The Paris Diet is fine for someone like you because it's extremely low in fat during the Weight Loss Program. On the Adjustment and Maintenance Programs, however, substitute a polyunsaturated margarine (made from corn or sunflower) for butter. Use monounsaturated oils, such as olive oil, along with those with a high polyunsaturated content, such as corn and sunflower oils. Naturally, you'll have to eliminate the yolks of eggs since they are high in cholesterol. Limit yourself to the low-fat dairy products recommended in our guidelines.

I've finally decided to stop smoking, but I'm scared of putting on weight. Can this program help me?

It certainly can. The nicotine in tobacco is an appetite suppressant and also burns up energy for reasons we don't yet fully understand. In other words, if a nonsmoker and a smoker eat the same number of calories, the smoker will put on less weight.

Unfortunately, when smokers quit they may put on weight even if they continue to eat the same amount of food as before. Things get even worse if extra food is substituted for the missing cigarettes: Some people have been known to put on as many as thirty pounds after quitting!

It's better to be safe than sorry. We recommend that you start the Paris Diet as soon as you stop smoking. If you're a woman who eats normally, start with Stage Two of the Adjustment Program; men can use Stages One or Two of the Maintenance Program. Stay on these diets for six to eight weeks. That should be sufficient time to allow your metabolism to adjust. Your energy intake and expenditure should reach the right balance at the end of this period.

You'll then be able to increase your food intake gradually, by following the Adjustment and Maintenance Programs. (Life-dieters should follow all four programs.) You may not lose weight, but you won't gain any either.

And by the way—congratulations for deciding to take that vital step toward better health.

I exercise in the gym three times a week for about an hour. Can I continue to do this while I'm on the diet?

You use up about 200 calories when you do a half hour workout at a reasonably fast pace. During the time you're on the Weight Loss Program, you won't be eating more than 900 calories a day. If you continue to exercise heavily, your body can't get enough energy to fill its needs. Therefore, take a vacation from the gym during these weeks. Instead, do ten to twenty minutes of light exercise at home by following the program in Chapter 12. Or you might walk at a normal pace for a half hour each day.

When you go back to the gym for the remaining weeks of the diet, cut out heavy aerobics. Instead, ask an instructor to help you devise a regimen that concentrates on the muscles of the abdomen, thighs, and buttocks. On-the-mat calisthenics are good for toning; so are cycling and swimming. You also could choose to follow our full exercise plan, which was designed to complement the entire Paris Diet.

Will I have to stay on a strict diet for the rest of my life just to look slim?

Certainly not! Women stop losing weight even though they eat like birds because they've been dieting for too long.

The Paris Diet teaches you new and better eating habits that you can follow for life if you don't want to gain weight again. The amount of time you stay on the program depends on whether you have ten, twenty, thirty, or sixty pounds to lose. Although you'll definitely lose all the weight you need to, the heavier you are, the longer it will take.

Once you are down to your ideal weight, it's up to you. All you have to do is follow the Maintenance Program for as long as possible —a minimum of two months is best, and then eat sensibly according to the principles of the program.

Whatever you do, avoid the "yo-yo" syndrome—that's your best insurance against having to diet for life. Don't lose weight, gain it back, lose it again, and so on. Each time you go on a new diet, it becomes harder and harder to lose weight.

But as we've said many times, if you follow the Paris Diet to the letter and then simply eat balanced, healthy meals afterward, you'll never have to diet again.

I'm twenty pounds overweight and about to start the program. Tell me the truth—will I ever get my once-perfect figure back?

It would be a lie to tell you that everyone can lose weight and look like a teenager again. A lot of factors determine the final cosmetic result of dieting, and age is the major one. It's much easier to snap back into shape at twenty, when your skin is more elastic, than it is at fifty.

The amount of weight you need to lose will also have a considerable effect on how you look at the end of the program. The best results are obtained when you have no more than twenty pounds to shed. Beyond that, your skin might become slack in some places after you've lost the weight.

When people are really obese, the best bet after weight loss may be plastic surgery. For everyone else, nature can be helped along in various ways:

In the gym—select exercises that firm up the pectoral muscles, abdomen, and thighs.

Massages—apart from the fact that they make you feel good, they can also improve skin tone wherever there is slack flesh.

Creams—although they can't make you look younger, most moisturizers do improve the texture and elasticity of the skin.

How is the Paris plan different from other diets?

The Paris Diet is less a weight loss diet than a way to lose all your unwanted weight and then restructure your metabolism so that you can eat more and eat better than ever before without gaining a pound.

Few diets can make this claim, and those that do often don't tell the truth. With most other plans you lose weight as long as you follow their strict rules, but gain it back the minute you slip. Or you have to remain on a restricted food plan for the rest of your life. Worst of all, the majority of diets don't even work for many women because they are life-dieters and have altered their metabolisms by eating too little. They can't lose any weight unless they completely starve themselves and seriously endanger their health.

The Paris Diet promises that everyone will lose the weight they want—from the biggest eaters to those who nibble like birds. It is designed to suit every size, sex, and metabolic rate. It is also designed to be healthy and invigorating.

And finally, its greatest feature is, as you would expect from its name, the food you eat. The Standard Diet has simple yet delicious meals, and the Chef's Menu is a gourmet's treat; even at Stage One of the Weight Loss Program, the food is so appetizing you won't believe you're actually losing weight.

PART SEVEN

———— ⚜ ————

The Paris Diet
Recipes

Note: Calorie and protein counts
are per serving

CHAPTER 14

✦

The Chef's Recipes

Soup and Salads

TOMATO GAZPACHO
Gaspacho de Tomates

2 servings
PREPARATION TIME: 10 MIN

1 pound tomatoes, quartered	*1 small onion, quartered*
¾ cup yogurt	*2 drops Tabasco*
1 clove garlic	*2 sprigs dill*

In a blender or food processor, combine the tomatoes, yogurt, garlic, onion, and Tabasco; purée until smooth. Refrigerate for 30 minutes.
Serve garnished with dill sprigs. Makes about 3 cups.

CALORIES: 110   PROTEIN: 8 g

RAW VEGETABLE SALAD
Salade Maraîchère

2 servings
PREPARATION TIME: 10 MIN

2 small carrots, shredded
4 large radishes, quartered
½ cucumber, sliced
yogurt sauce (recipe page 249) or
   lemon juice

1 tsp fresh parsley, chopped
pepper, freshly ground

Arrange vegetables on serving plates.

Drizzle with yogurt sauce or lemon juice. Sprinkle with parsley and pepper.

with lemon juice

CALORIES: 20   PROTEIN: 0.5 g

with yogurt sauce

CALORIES: 47   PROTEIN: 3 g

MIXED VEGETABLE SALAD
Salade Marignan

2 servings
PREPARATION TIME: 10–15 MIN

1 medium carrot, peeled and sliced
1 small turnip, peeled and thinly
  sliced
1 cup green beans, trimmed
½ cup cauliflower
½ cup broccoli
1 medium zucchini, sliced

¼ cup chopped chervil or basil
2 plum tomatoes or 1 medium-size
  tomato, quartered
1 tbs sherry or balsamic vinegar
2 cups mixed salad greens
1 tsp chopped coriander or parsley

Place carrots, turnips, and beans in a vegetable steamer over boiling water; cover and steam for 2 minutes. Add cauliflower, broccoli, and zucchini and steam 4 minutes more. Cool.

In a blender or food processor, combine chervil, tomatoes, and vinegar; blend until smooth.

Place salad greens in the middle of each plate; put the vegetables around it. Drizzle with the tomato sauce, and sprinkle with coriander.

CALORIES: 62   PROTEIN: 5 g

SPRINGTIME GREEN BEAN SALAD
Salade de Haricots Verts Printanière

2 servings

PREPARATION TIME: ABOUT 15 MIN

1½ cups green beans, trimmed	*1 tbs fresh parsley, chopped*
1 cup broccoli	*2 tsp lemon juice*
1 tbs olive oil	*1 tsp fresh chives, chopped*
1 tbs wine vinegar	*1 cup curly endive*
1 tbs mustard	*½ cup mushrooms, thinly sliced*

Place green beans in vegetable steamer; steam over boiling water 4 minutes. Add broccoli and steam 2 minutes more. Rinse under cool water and drain.

Combine oil, vinegar, mustard, parsley, lemon juice, and chives; whisk until blended.

Arrange the endive on two plates. Arrange green beans, broccoli, and mushroom slices around it. Drizzle with dressing.

Recommendation for the wine: A white Loire valley wine or a Burgundy (if permitted on plan).

CALORIES: 97   PROTEIN: 4 g

Sauces, Dressings, and Condiments

RED VINAIGRETTE
Vinaigre Zéro

12 1 tbs servings or ¾ cup
PREPARATION TIME: 5 MIN

½ cup tomato juice
1 tbs lemon juice or cider vinegar
1 tbs onion, finely chopped
1 tbs parsley, chives, or coriander,
   finely chopped

1 tsp Dijon mustard
¼ tsp paprika
⅛ tsp pepper, freshly ground

In a small bowl, combine all ingredients; mix until blended. Cover and refrigerate up to 1 week.

CALORIES: 1   PROTEIN: 0 g

VINAIGRETTE WITH TARRAGON
Sauce Provençale

12 1 tbs servings or ¾ cup
PREPARATION TIME: 3 MIN

1 tbs Dijon mustard
¼ cup balsamic vinegar
2 tbs water
2 tbs fresh lemon juice
¼ tsp tarragon, dried or fresh

1 clove garlic, finely minced
salt and freshly ground pepper to
taste
¼ cup safflower oil

Combine all ingredients, except oil, in blender or food processor and blend. Gradually add oil until mixture thickens. Chill well before serving.

CALORIES: 37   PROTEIN: 0.1 g

MINT VINEGAR
Sauce Menthe

4 1 tbs servings or ¼ cup
PREPARATION TIME: 10 MIN

¼ cup fresh mint, chopped
¾ cup white vinegar
3 tbs water

salt and freshly ground pepper to
taste

With the edge of a wooden spoon, bruise mint leaves. Boil vinegar and reduce to 2 tablespoons. Add mint, water, salt, and pepper. Bring to boil for 5 minutes. Strain through fine sieve and discard leaves.

CALORIES: 5   PROTEIN: 0 g

YOGURT SAUCE
Sauce Yogourt

8 1 tbs servings or ½ cup
PREPARATION TIME: 3 MIN

½ cup plain low-fat yogurt
1 tsp fresh parsley, finely chopped
1 tsp Dijon mustard

¼ clove garlic, finely chopped
1 small pickle, finely chopped
pepper, freshly ground

In a small bowl, combine all ingredients. Whisk until blended. Cover and refrigerate up to 1 week.

CALORIES: 7   PROTEIN: 0.7 g

CREAMY SPINACH DRESSING
Sauce Sontay

24 1 tbs servings or 1½ cups
PREPARATION TIME: 5 MIN

¼ cup fresh parsley, chopped
¼ cup fresh or frozen spinach, chopped
1 tbs fresh dill, chopped, or 1 tsp dried

1 clove garlic (optional)
1 cup plain low-fat yogurt
cayenne pepper to taste
salt and black pepper to taste

Place all ingredients in a blender or food processor and combine thoroughly. Adjust seasoning. Chill well.

CALORIES: 6   PROTEIN: 0.6 g

CREAMED GARLIC DRESSING
Sauce Aïoli

12 1 tbs servings or ¾ cup
PREPARATION TIME: 3 MIN

½ cup evaporated skim milk
2 tbs fresh lemon juice
2 large cloves garlic, minced
1 tsp dried basil

¼ tsp paprika
¼ tsp white pepper
1 tsp olive oil
dash cayenne pepper

Place all ingredients in blender or food processor, and blend until smooth. Chill well and adjust seasonings before serving.

CALORIES: 7   PROTEIN: 0.5 g

WATERCRESS DRESSING
Sauce Grande Bêche

32 1 tbs servings or 2 cups
PREPARATION TIME: 3 MIN

1 cup watercress leaves, thoroughly
   washed and drained
½ cup low-calorie ricotta cheese
⅔ cup buttermilk
3 tbs scallion, chopped

1 tbs anchovy paste
½ cup fresh lemon juice
¼ tsp tarragon, dried or fresh
salt and freshly ground pepper to
   taste

In a food processor or blender, pulse watercress leaves several times until chopped. Add remaining ingredients, and process until blended.

CALORIES: 9   PROTEIN: 0.7 g

PIPERADE DRESSING
Sauce Saint-Jeannet

24 1 tbs servings or 1½ cups
PREPARATION TIME: 3 MIN

½ red bell pepper, cored, seeded,
  and chopped (approx. ½ cup)
½ fresh tomato, diced (approx.
  ¼ cup)
2 fresh basil leaves, chopped, or
  ½ tsp dried
2 tbs onion, chopped
½ tsp dried tarragon

dash red pepper flakes or cayenne
  pepper (optional)
salt and freshly ground pepper to
  taste
2 tsp balsamic vinegar
1 tsp olive oil
½ cup buttermilk

Place all ingredients, except buttermilk, in a food processor or blender, and purée until smooth. Add buttermilk and process until blended. Chill.

CALORIES: 5   PROTEIN: 0.3 g

GREEN DRESSING
Sauce Verte

24 1 tbs servings or 1 1/2 cups
PREPARATION TIME: 4 MIN

1/4 cup fresh parsley, chopped
1/4 cup fresh or frozen spinach,
  chopped
1 tbs fresh dill, chopped, or 1 tsp
  dried

1 clove garlic (optional)
1 cup plain low-fat yogurt
cayenne pepper to taste
salt and freshly ground black pepper
  to taste

Place all ingredients in a blender or food processor, and combine thoroughly. Adjust seasonings. Chill well.

Variation: Eliminate spinach and dill. Add 1/4 cup chopped chives and juice of 1/2 lemon.

CALORIES: 6   PROTEIN: 0.6 g

ROQUEFORT CHEESE DRESSING
Sauce Roquefort

24 1 tbs servings or 1 1/2 cups
PREPARATION TIME: 3 MIN

1/4 cup Roquefort cheese, crumbled
1/2 cup plain low-fat yogurt
1/2 cup buttermilk

1/2 clove garlic
dash cayenne pepper (optional)
black pepper, freshly ground, to taste

Place all ingredients in blender or food processor, and process until well blended. Refrigerate until chilled.

CALORIES: 9   PROTEIN: 0.7 g

SPICY TOMATO SAUCE
Sauce Tomates aux Aromates

2 servings
PREPARATION TIME: 5 MIN

½ cup tomato juice
½ stalk celery, finely chopped
2 tsp green onion, thinly sliced
1 tsp fresh lemon juice

2 drops Worcestershire sauce
1 small clove garlic, finely chopped
pinch ground nutmeg
pinch pepper, freshly ground

In a small bowl, combine all ingredients and mix thoroughly. Cover and refrigerate up to 1 week.

CALORIES: 19   PROTEIN: 0.9 g

TOMATO AND LEMON SAUCE WITH HERBS
Sauce Maraîchère

2 servings
PREPARATION TIME: 5 MIN

½ cup tomato juice
3 tbs lemon juice
1 tsp plain low-fat yogurt
½ tsp fresh parsley, finely chopped

½ tsp fresh coriander, finely chopped
¼ tsp fresh thyme
pinch pepper, freshly ground
pinch artificial sweetener

In a small bowl, combine all ingredients; mix until well blended. Cover and refrigerate up to 1 week.

CALORIES: 19   PROTEIN: 1 g

CHINESE-STYLE TOMATO SAUCE
Sauce Tomates à la Chinoise

2 servings
PREPARATION TIME: 5 MIN

½ cup tomato juice   ½ tsp low-sodium soy sauce
½ tsp red wine vinegar

In a small bowl, combine all ingredients; mix until blended. Cover
and refrigerate up to 2 weeks.

CALORIES: 15   PROTEIN: 1 g

ONION PRESERVE
WITH GRENADINE
Confiture d'Oignons Grenadine

2 servings
PREPARATION TIME: 15 MIN

1 tbs olive oil   2 tbs grenadine syrup
1 lb onions, sliced   ¼ tsp pepper, freshly ground

Heat the oil in a large skillet. Add the onions, and cook over medium
high heat until translucent, about 10 minutes. Stir in the grenadine
syrup and pepper, and cook 5 minutes over low heat.
    Serve with grilled meats or as a vegetable.

CALORIES: 217   PROTEIN: 2 g

Vegetables

DUET OF ASPARAGUS AND MUSHROOMS
Asperges aux Champignons en Duo

2 servings
PREPARATION TIME: 15 MIN

8 asparagus spears, trimmed
2 cups mixed salad greens (escarole,
   radicchio, wild chicory, lamb's
   lettuce, dandelion, watercress,
   arugula), rinsed

1 cup white mushrooms, sliced
2 tbs plain low-fat yogurt
1 tsp Dijon mustard
1 tsp lemon juice
pepper, freshly ground

Heat 1-inch water to boiling in a medium skillet over high heat. Add asparagus spears, and cook until just tender, about 5 minutes. Rinse under cool water; drain. Arrange greens on each serving plate. Top with asparagus spears and mushroom slices.

In a small bowl combine yogurt, Dijon mustard, and lemon juice; stir until blended. Drizzle over vegetables, and season with pepper.

CALORIES: 65   PROTEIN: 6 g

BROCCOLI SOUFFLÉ WITH TWO SPICES
Soufflé de Brocolis aux Deux Épices

2 servings
PREPARATION TIME: 15 MIN

2½ cups broccoli

2 egg whites

1 tsp fresh coriander, chopped

1 tsp fresh marjoram, chopped

⅛ tsp pepper

Preheat oven to 375 degrees.

Place the broccoli in a vegetable steamer. Cover and steam over boiling water for about 5 minutes. Rinse and cool broccoli, then finely chop it.

In a bowl whip egg whites until soft peaks form. Fold in chopped broccoli, coriander, marjoram, and pepper. Scoop into a 2-cup gratin dish or two 1 cup soufflé dishes. Bake 10 to 15 minutes until golden and puffed.

CALORIES: 46   PROTEIN: 7 g

SLICED CARROTS WITH PARSLEY
Carottes Vichy

2 servings

PREPARATION TIME: 10 MIN

2 cups carrots, sliced
½ cup water

pinch pepper, freshly ground
1 tsp fresh parsley, chopped

In a small saucepan, combine carrots with water and pepper. Cover and bring to a boil; reduce heat and simmer about 5 minutes, until tender and most of the liquid is evaporated. Drain and sprinkle with parsley.

CALORIES: 46   PROTEIN: 1 g

CARROT CAKES
WITH ASPARAGUS SAUCE
Gâteau de Carottes au Coulis d'Asperges

2 servings
PREPARATION TIME: 25 MIN

3 cups carrots, shredded (about
   12 oz)
2 cups low-sodium chicken broth
2 eggs

1 tbs chervil or parsley, chopped
⅛ tsp pepper, freshly ground
8 oz fresh or canned asparagus
2 tbs plain low-fat yogurt

Preheat oven to 350 degrees.

Combine carrots and chicken broth in a medium saucepan; bring to a boil and cook until carrots are tender. Drain carrots (reserving ¼ cup liquid), pressing out any excess liquid.

In a bowl, beat eggs, chervil, and pepper; stir in carrots. Fill two 1-cup molds with mixture; place in a shallow baking pan. Fill pan halfway up sides of molds with warm water. Cover each mold with foil, and bake 15 minutes. Uncover and bake 5 minutes more or until centers are set.

Meanwhile, fill a medium skillet with 1 inch of water; heat to boiling. Add asparagus and cook until tender, 6–8 minutes. Cut tips from asparagus and reserve. In blender or food processor, combine asparagus spears, reserved liquid, yogurt and peppers. Purée until smooth.

Unmold carrot cakes onto serving plates; top with asparagus sauce and reserved asparagus tips.

CALORIES: 209   PROTEIN: 14 g

PROVENCE-STYLE TOMATOES
Tomates Provençale

2 servings
PREPARATION TIME: 10 MIN

2 tsp parsley, finely chopped
2 tsp coriander, finely chopped
1 clove garlic, finely chopped

pinch pepper, freshly ground
2 tomatoes, halved

Preheat broiler.

Combine herbs, garlic, and pepper. Arrange tomato halves, cut sides up, on broiler tray and sprinkle with herb mixture. Broil 3 inches from heat for 3 minutes.

CALORIES: 40

PROTEIN: 2 g

STUFFED ZUCCHINI
Courgettes Farcies

2 servings
PREPARATION TIME: 40 MIN

1 tbs onion, finely chopped	*2 medium zucchini*
1 tbs parsley, finely chopped	*2 oz lean ground beef*
1 tbs coriander, finely chopped	*1 tbs Parmesan or Swiss cheese,*
¼ cup tomato juice	*grated*
¼ cup water	*⅛ tsp pepper, freshly ground*

Preheat oven to 400 degrees.

In a small skillet, sauté onion, parsley, and coriander for 1 minute over medium heat. Add tomato juice and water and heat to boiling; reduce heat and simmer 5 minutes.

Meanwhile, cut each zucchini in half length-wise and hollow out each half with a small spoon. Chop pulp finely. In a small bowl, combine beef, cheese, pepper, and chopped zucchini. Fill each zucchini shell with this mixture. Arrange stuffed zucchini in a shallow baking dish. Pour tomato sauce over zucchini and bake 25–30 minutes.

CALORIES: 122   PROTEIN: 10 g

ZUCCHINI WITH MEAT STUFFING
Courgettes Farcies à la Viande

2 servings
PREPARATION TIME: 30 MIN

2 medium zucchini
1 cup (4 oz) leftover cooked chicken,
   chopped
¼ cup onion, chopped
1 tbs parsley, chopped

½ tsp fresh tarragon or thyme,
   chopped
⅛ tsp pepper, freshly ground
2 plum tomatoes, halved length-wise
   and sliced

Preheat oven to 400 degrees.

Cut each zucchini in half length-wise; hollow out with a teaspoon.

In a small bowl, combine chicken, onion, parsley, tarragon, and pepper. Arrange zucchini halves in a shallow baking dish. Fill each zucchini with meat mixture. Arrange tomato slices on top of filling. Bake 20 minutes.

You can also use the stuffing for tomatoes, peppers, or small eggplants.

CALORIES: 172   PROTEIN: 15 g

ZUCCHINI WITH PINK SHRIMP
Courgettes aux Crevettes Roses

2 servings
PREPARATION TIME: 15 MIN

2 medium zucchini
4 oz cooked shrimp
2 tbs yogurt sauce (recipe
  page 249)

lettuce leaves
2 lemon wedges

Cut each zucchini in half, length-wise. Scoop out the insides with a teaspoon. Drop the zucchini shells into boiling water until barely tender. Drain well.

Arrange lettuce leaves on each plate. Place 2 zucchini halves on each plate. Fill the zucchini with shrimp and cover with the yogurt sauce.

Serve with lemon wedges.

CALORIES: 78   PROTEIN: 12 g

STEWED VEGETABLES
MEDITERRANEAN STYLE
Ratatouille

2 servings

PREPARATION TIME: 50 MIN

1 medium zucchini, sliced	1 medium onion, finely chopped
1 medium eggplant, sliced	fresh thyme sprigs
2 tomatoes, quartered	1 bay leaf
half a green pepper, cut in thin strips	½ cup water

In a large nonstick saucepan layer vegetables, placing a thyme sprig between each layer. Add a bay leaf and water. Cover and bring to a boil. Reduce heat and simmer 40 minutes or until vegetables are very tender. If vegetables begin to stick, add water by ¼ cups.

CALORIES: 71   PROTEIN: 3 g

VEGETABLE ASPIC
WITH TOMATO SAUCE
Aspic de Légumes au Coulis de Tomates

2 servings
PREPARATION TIME: 20 MIN PLUS CHILLING

2 carrots, halved length-wise then
   quartered
2 cups low-sodium chicken broth
4 oz green beans, trimmed (about
   18 beans)
½ cup frozen peas

1 envelope unflavored gelatin
¼ cup cold water
fresh basil leaves
2 tomatoes, quartered
pepper, freshly ground, to taste

Place carrots and chicken broth in a medium saucepan; heat to boiling. Reduce heat and cook until carrots are tender, about 7 minutes. With a slotted spoon, remove carrots and set aside. Add green beans to broth; cover and cook until tender, about 6 minutes. With a slotted spoon, remove beans and set aside. Add peas and cook 2 minutes. With a slotted spoon, remove peas and set aside. Reserve broth.

Meanwhile, in a small saucepan sprinkle the gelatin over ¼ cup water; set aside.

Over low heat, warm gelatin until granules are dissolved. Add broth to gelatin.

In a 4-cup ring or other mold, arrange basil leaves and vegetables in an attractive pattern. Pour broth mixture over; cover and refrigerate at least 4 hours.

Meanwhile, place tomatoes in food processor or blender and pulse with on/off motion until chunky. Season with freshly ground pepper.

When gelatin has set, dip for a couple of seconds in warm water to release mold. Invert and serve with tomato sauce.

CALORIES: 117   PROTEIN: 9 g

Meats

OLD-FASHIONED FILET OF BEEF
Filet de Boeuf Grand-Mère

2 servings
PREPARATION TIME: 20 MIN

2 medium carrots, cut julienne
1 cup (4 oz) leeks, sliced
1 small (2 oz) celery stalk, sliced
3 cups water

2 slices of lean filet mignon, 4 oz
   each
pepper, freshly ground

In a medium saucepan, combine the vegetables and water; bring to a boil over high heat. Reduce heat and simmer about 10 minutes. Remove the vegetables with a slotted spoon. Add the filet mignon and simmer to desired readiness, about 5 minutes for medium rare. Place beef in soup plates and serve with some of the vegetables and broth. Season with pepper and serve.

CALORIES: 220   PROTEIN: 24 g

BEEF FILET WITH SPICES
Coeur de Filet de Boeuf aux Épices

2 servings
PREPARATION TIME: 15 MIN

2 cups green beans
2 beef filet steaks, 5 oz each

1 tbs mixed peppercorns, (crushed
black, white, pink, and green
peppercorns), coarsely ground

Place the green beans in a vegetable steamer and steam 6–8 minutes, until tender.

Meanwhile, roll the 2 beef filets in the crushed peppercorns. Heat a heavy skillet over high heat. Add filets and sear 2–3 minutes per side for medium rare.

Serve with the green beans.

CALORIES: 270   PROTEIN: 30 g

BEEF FILETS WITH SHALLOTS
Filets de Boeuf aux Échalotes

2 servings
PREPARATION TIME: 15 MIN

2 beef filet steaks (5½ oz each)
pepper, freshly ground
2 shallots, sliced
½ cup red wine

1 tsp butter
1 cup carrots, sliced
1 cup cauliflower

Season steaks with pepper. Heat a heavy skillet over medium high heat. Coat with vegetable cooking spray, and cook steaks 3–4 minutes per side for medium rare. Remove steaks and keep warm; add shallots to skillet and cook 2 minutes. Add wine, stirring to scrape up any meat drippings, and cook 3 minutes or until wine is reduced by half. Stir in butter and serve with meat.

As the meat cooks, place carrots in vegetable steamer and steam 4 minutes. Add cauliflower and steam 3–4 minutes more. Serve vegetables with beef.

CALORIES: 335   PROTEIN: 37 g

SAUTÉED VEAL
WITH SMALL VEGETABLES
Sauté de Veau aux Petits Légumes

2 servings
PREPARATION TIME: 10 MIN

2 cups carrots, sliced	1 tsp olive oil
1 onion, sliced	8 oz veal cutlets
¼ tsp fresh thyme	½ lemon, sliced
1 bay leaf	¼ cup water

Place carrots, onion, thyme, and bay leaf in a vegetable steamer. Steam over boiling water about 6 minutes, until carrots are tender.

Meanwhile, heat a medium nonstick skillet over medium high heat. Add olive oil. When hot, add cutlets and sauté about 1 minute on each side. Remove cutlets and keep warm. Add lemon slices and water and cook 2 minutes. Pour over veal and serve with steamed vegetables.

CALORIES: 204   PROTEIN: 25 g

VEAL CUTLETS WITH SAGE
Émincé de Veau à la Sauge

2 servings
PREPARATION TIME: 10 MIN

3 cloves garlic, quartered
6 sage leaves
2 tbs water

8 oz veal cutlets
¼ cup dry white wine

Heat a nonstick skillet over low heat; add garlic and sauté 1 minute. Add sage leaves and water; cook until water evaporates. Remove garlic and sage; set aside. Increase heat to medium. Add veal and sauté 3 minutes, turning once. Remove veal from pan; keep warm. Add wine to skillet; increase heat to high and boil 2 minutes. Pour over veal and garnish with garlic and sage.

CALORIES: 198

PROTEIN: 24 g

LAMB WITH MIXED VEGETABLES
Croquette d'Agneau en Bouquet de Légumes

2 servings
PREPARATION TIME: 20 MIN

2 loin lamb chops, well trimmed | 2 plum tomatoes, sliced
(about 10–12 oz) | ½ tsp fresh thyme
1 clove garlic, halved | pepper, freshly ground
2 cups white mushrooms, sliced | 2 lemon wedges
1 medium zucchini, thinly sliced

Rub each side of lamb chops with garlic; set aside.

On each salad plate, arrange mushrooms in center. Surround with a circle of zucchini slices. Arrange a circle of tomato slices at outer edge. Cover each plate with plastic wrap; pierce to vent plastic.

Heat a heavy skillet over high heat. Microwave vegetable plates on high for 3 minutes; let stand covered 2 minutes. Meanwhile, add lamb chops to skillet and cook 2–3 minutes per side for medium rare. Serve with vegetables and a lemon wedge.

CALORIES: 428   PROTEIN: 29 g

PORK TENDERLOIN
WITH EGGPLANT
Porc Colombo

2 servings
PREPARATION TIME: 15 MIN

*1 small eggplant, sliced in 1/4-inch
rounds
1 clove garlic, minced
1/2 tsp fresh thyme, chopped
pinch ground cloves*

*10 oz pork tenderloin, sliced 1/2-inch
thick
2 tbs lime juice
1/4 cup water*

Preheat broiler. Line broiler tray with aluminum foil, and spray with
vegetable cooking spray. Arrange eggplant slices on foil and broil
about 3 minutes per side, until tender and browned.

Meanwhile, combine garlic, thyme, and clove; rub on pork slices.
Heat a large skillet over medium high heat. Add pork and sauté 2
minutes per side. Remove pork from skillet and keep warm. Add
lime juice and water to skillet, stirring to scrape up any drippings
from the meat. Cook 2 minutes. Arrange a circle of eggplant slices
on each plate; top with pork and serve with lime sauce.

CALORIES: 317   PROTEIN: 42 g

MIXED GRILLED MEAT
Panaché de Viande Grillée

2 servings

PREPARATION TIME: 55–60 MIN

3 oz veal cutlet   1 medium tomato, chopped
3 oz beef tenderloin   ¼ cup red onion, chopped
3 oz pork tenderloin   ½ green pepper, chopped
2 cups water   1 tsp chervil or parsley, chopped
½ cup wild rice

Slice all meat about ¼-inch thick; refrigerate.

Bring water to boiling in a medium saucepan; add wild rice and cook 45 minutes. Stir in tomato, red onion, and green pepper, and cook 10 minutes more, until rice is tender. Add vegetables to rice and set aside, keeping warm. Preheat broiler or grill. Arrange rack as close as possible to heat source. Grill meat slices about 30 seconds per side. Sprinkle with chervil or parsley. Serve with the wild rice.

CALORIES: 366   PROTEIN: 32 g

Poultry

CHICKEN BREASTS
WITH CUCUMBER SPAGHETTI
Blanc de Volaille aux Spaghetti de Concombre

2 servings
PREPARATION TIME: 20 MIN

half a medium cucumber, seeded and
   cut into matchsticks
1 tsp vegetable oil
2 (9 oz) boneless, skinless chicken
   breasts, split

3 tbs water
1 tsp light cream
salt and pepper, to taste

In a small saucepan, boil the cucumber for about 2 minutes in water, then remove and cool under running water; drain and set aside.

Heat oil into a small skillet over medium high heat. Season chicken breasts with salt and pepper and cook for 3 minutes on each side. Remove the meat. Pour off any excess fat from pan then add water; heat to boiling. Remove from heat and stir in cream. Arrange the cucumber spaghetti in a circle on plate. Place the chicken in the center and cover with sauce.

CALORIES: 236   PROTEIN: 32 g

CHICKEN BREASTS WITH BROCCOLI AND CAULIFLOWER
Émincé de Volaille aux Deux Choux

2 servings
PREPARATION TIME: 15 MIN

1 cup low-sodium chicken broth
2 (9 oz) boneless skinless chicken
* breast halves*

1 tsp light cream
2 cups broccoli flowerets
2 cups cauliflowerets

In a small skillet, bring the chicken broth to a boil. Reduce heat and add chicken breasts. Cover and simmer 10 minutes. Remove chicken and keep warm. Cook the broth over high heat until it is reduced to about ¼ cup. Stir in cream.

Meanwhile, place the broccoli and cauliflowerets in a vegetable steamer; steam over boiling water 5 minutes or just until tender.

Slice chicken breasts into thin slices. Arrange chicken breasts in the center of the plate, with the warm vegetables around it. Spoon sauce over the whole dish.

CALORIES: 281   PROTEIN: 40 g

CHICKEN FLAVORED
WITH TRUFFLES
Jambonnette de Volaille au Parfum de Truffes

2 servings
PREPARATION TIME: 30 MIN

1 tbs truffles, finely chopped, or
  ¼ cup wild mushrooms such as
  shiitakes, finely chopped
2 chicken breast cutlets (9 oz),
  pounded ¼-inch thick

pepper, freshly ground
1 tsp olive oil
1¼ cups green beans
1 carrot, thinly sliced
1 medium zucchini, thinly sliced

Spread half the chopped truffles (or mushrooms) on one half of each chicken cutlet. Fold other half over filling; secure with toothpicks. Season with pepper.

Heat oil in a small skillet over medium high heat. Cook cutlets 4 minutes; turn and cook 4 minutes more. Meanwhile, place green beans and carrot slices in vegetable steamer; steam over boiling water 5 minutes. Add zucchini and steam 3 minutes more. Serve chicken with vegetables.

CALORIES: 166   PROTEIN: 24 g

TARRAGON-FLAVORED CHICKEN
Pilon de Volaille Cuit aux Senteurs d'Estragon

2 servings
PREPARATION TIME: 30 MIN

1 (9 oz) boneless skinless chicken breast, split	1 cup wild mushrooms, such as morels, shiitakes, sliced
1 tsp fresh tarragon, chopped	¼ cup low-sodium chicken broth
½ tsp butter	1 tsp light cream
2 cups fresh broccoli	

Rub the chicken with half the tarragon.

In a small skillet over medium high heat, melt butter.

Add chicken and sauté 5 minutes on each side.

Meanwhile, arrange broccoli in steamer basket in saucepan; cover and cook 3 minutes.

Remove chicken from pan; transfer to serving plate and keep warm. Add mushrooms and cook 3 minutes. Scoop onto chicken. Add chicken broth and remaining tarragon to skillet and boil 2 minutes. Remove from heat and stir in cream. Pour over chicken and mushrooms, and serve immediately.

CALORIES: 242   PROTEIN: 38 g

TRUFFLE-FLAVORED CHICKEN CASSEROLE

Poularde en Cocotte aux Senteurs de Truffes

2 servings

PREPARATION TIME: 30 MIN

2 (9 oz) boneless skinless chicken
    breast halves
1 tsp black truffle slivers
½ cup carrots, sliced
1 small turnip, thinly sliced

1 small onion, thinly sliced
1 cup white mushrooms, sliced
1 celery stalk, thinly sliced
1 cup water

With a thin knife, make small slits in each chicken breast; stuff with truffle slivers.

Place all the vegetables and water in a pressure cooker. Arrange chicken on top. Seal pressure cooker according to instructions, and cook over high heat until valve pops up. Reduce heat to medium and cook 10 minutes. Open pressure cooker carefully. Serve chicken with the vegetables.

CALORIES: 239

PROTEIN: 30 g

BREADED CHICKEN
WITH SESAME SEEDS
Poulet Pané au Sésame

2 servings

PREPARATION TIME: 15 MIN

1 tbs plain low-fat yogurt
1 tsp Dijon mustard
1 tsp Gruyère or Parmesan cheese,
  grated

1 tsp sesame seeds, crushed
⅛ tsp pepper, freshly ground
2 (9 oz) boneless skinless chicken
  breast halves

Preheat oven to 450 degrees.

On a flat plate, combine all ingredients except chicken; stir until blended. Dip the chicken pieces in the mustard mixture.

Arrange the chicken on a foil-lined baking sheet, and bake 10 minutes or until juices run clear when chicken is pierced.

CALORIES: 254   PROTEIN: 37 g

TANDOORI CHICKEN
Poulet Tandoori

2 servings
PREPARATION TIME: 45 MIN PLUS MARINATING

1 (9 oz) skinless chicken breast, split	*1 tsp ground ginger*
½ cup plain low-fat yogurt	*1 tsp paprika*
1 tbs lemon juice	*⅛ tsp pepper, freshly ground*
1 clove garlic, chopped	*2 lemon wedges*
1 tsp curry powder	

Make shallow gashes in chicken to allow the marinade to penetrate. In a shallow baking dish, combine remaining ingredients except lemon wedges and stir until blended. Add the chicken pieces, turning several times to coat thoroughly. Marinate 30 minutes or cover and marinate in the refrigerator overnight.

Preheat oven to 450 degrees.

Line a baking sheet with foil; arrange chicken pieces on foil. Bake 35–40 minutes or until juices run clear when chicken is pierced. Serve with lemon wedges.

CALORIES: 242   PROTEIN: 34 g

STEWED CHICKEN BASQUE STYLE
Poulet Basquaise

2 servings
PREPARATION TIME: 1 HOUR

1 onion, chopped
1 green pepper, coarsely chopped
1 lb tomatoes, coarsely chopped, or
  1 can (16 oz) whole tomatoes,
  chopped

1 clove garlic, chopped
2 whole chicken legs, skin removed
pepper, freshly ground

In a large saucepan combine onion, green pepper, tomatoes, garlic, and chicken. Season with pepper. Heat mixture to boiling then reduce heat and simmer, half covered, 45–50 minutes or until chicken is tender.

CALORIES: 282   PROTEIN: 35 g

CHICKEN BAKED
IN A SALT CRUST
Poulet en Croûte de Sel

6 servings

PREPARATION TIME: 1½ HOURS

4 cups all-purpose flour
4 cups kosher salt
2 eggs

1¼ to 1½ cups water
1 3-pound roasting chicken, patted
dry

Preheat oven to 450 degrees.

Line a large Dutch oven (large enough to hold the chicken) with 2 sheets of aluminum foil placed perpendicular so that the foil overhangs the sides of the Dutch oven by about 10 inches in each direction.

In a large mixing bowl, combine flour and salt. Beat one of the eggs with 1¼ cups of water; add to dry ingredients and stir to form a shapeable dough, adding remaining ¼ cup water if necessary.

Between 2 sheets of lightly floured wax paper, roll dough to ⅛-inch thickness. Remove top sheet of wax paper and place chicken on dough. Bring dough up over chicken and pinch edges to enclose completely. Place chicken in the Dutch oven. Beat remaining egg and brush over dough.

Wrap foil over chicken to enclose completely. Bake chicken for 1¼ hours.

To serve, remove chicken from foil and break open salt crust. Do not eat crust.

CALORIES: 212   PROTEIN: 36 g

CHICKEN SALAD
WITH WHISKEY DRESSING
Fondant de Volaille au Whisky

2 servings
PREPARATION TIME: 20 MIN PLUS COOLING

*1–2 boneless skinless chicken
  breast(s) (9 oz)*
2 cups water
½ cup tomatoes, diced
½ cup celery, sliced
½ cup green pepper, diced
4 romaine lettuce leaves, shredded

DRESSING
¼ cup plain low-fat yogurt
1 tbs low-calorie mayonnaise
1½ tsp whiskey or bourbon
¼ tsp pepper

In a medium saucepan, cover the chicken breasts with water. Heat just to boiling, then reduce heat and poach breasts for 10 minutes.

Meanwhile, make the dressing: Combine all ingredients in a small bowl and stir until smooth.

Remove chicken from saucepan and allow to cool completely. Cut in large cubes. Combine chicken, tomatoes, celery, and green pepper with dressing in a bowl and toss to coat. Add the whiskey.

Serve on a bed of shredded romaine lettuce.

CALORIES: 257   PROTEIN: 43 g

DUCK SLIVERS
WITH TWO PEPPERS
Émincé de Canard aux Deux Poivres

2 servings
PREPARATION TIME: 30 MIN

1 tsp vegetable oil
11 oz boneless skinless duck breast
2 tbs water
1 tbs wine vinegar
½ tsp white pepper, crushed

½ tsp black pepper, crushed
1 packet artificial sweetener
1 tbs Dijon mustard
½ cup orzo pasta, cooked according
to instructions

Heat oil in a nonstick skillet over high heat. Sauté the duck breast 2 minutes on each side; transfer to a plate. Add water and wine vinegar to skillet; bring to a boil. Add the white and black crushed pepper and artificial sweetener; cook 30 seconds. Add the mustard and any juices from the duck; cover to keep warm.

Cut the duck breast in thin slices; arrange the slices on each plate. Spoon sauce over meat. Serve with cooked pasta.

CALORIES: 553   PROTEIN: 45 g

TURKEY FILET
IN FRENCH ACADEMY COSTUME
Filet de Dinde en Habit-Vert

2 servings
PREPARATION TIME: 20 MIN

4 leaves green cabbage
¾ cup small young carrots
1 tsp vegetable oil
11 oz turkey breast filet
2 tbs wine vinegar

2 tbs water
2 tbs catsup
1 tbs grainy mustard (Moutarde de
  Meaux)

In a medium saucepan, steam the cabbage leaves for 4 minutes over boiling water; remove. Add the carrots to the pan of water and simmer until tender, about 5 minutes.

Meanwhile, pour vegetable oil into a medium-size skillet, and sauté the turkey filets 2 minutes on each side. Remove meat to a plate. Add wine vinegar and water to skillet; heat to boiling. Add catsup and any juices from the meat.

Coat each turkey filet with the mustard, then wrap in a cabbage leaf. Place in the center of each plate, arrange the carrots around it, and cover the whole dish with the catsup sauce.

CALORIES: 346   PROTEIN: 46 g

TURKEY SUPREME IN PAPILLOTES
Suprême de Dinde en Papillotes

2 servings
PREPARATION TIME: 25 MIN

9 oz turkey breast filet
pepper, freshly ground
1 tbs truffle juice or ½ tsp fresh
   rosemary or thyme, chopped

2 cups broccoli
8 cherry tomatoes

Preheat oven to 400 degrees.

Coat a medium skillet with vegetable cooking spray. Heat over high heat. Add turkey breast and sear 30 seconds on each side.

Fold a 14-inch sheet of aluminum foil in half cross-wise. Open foil and place turkey on one half. Season with pepper, and sprinkle with truffle juice or herbs. Crimp ends of foil to enclose turkey completely. Bake 10 minutes.

After turkey has been baking 5 minutes, place broccoli in a vegetable steamer; steam 3 minutes over boiling water. Add cherry tomatoes and steam 2 minutes more.

To serve turkey, slit the foil and open carefully.

CALORIES: 240

PROTEIN: 40 g

Eggs

SCRAMBLED EGGS WITH TOMATOES AND SWEET PEPPERS
Piperade

2 servings
PREPARATION TIME: 25 MIN

2 tomatoes, cut in 1-inch chunks or
   14 oz can tomatoes, drained and
   chopped
½ green pepper, cut in ½-inch
   chunks

1 small clove garlic, chopped
2 eggs plus 2 egg whites
pepper, freshly ground

Place tomatoes, green pepper, and garlic in a large nonstick skillet. Cover and cook 15 minutes over medium heat. Increase heat to medium high; uncover and cook 5 minutes more to allow some of the liquid to evaporate.

Meanwhile, beat the eggs and egg whites together in a small bowl. Season with pepper. Add the eggs to the skillet, and cook 3–4 minutes more. Texture will be lumpy.

You may cook the eggs separately in a small nonstick skillet and serve the piperade sauce separately.

CALORIES: 120   PROTEIN: 11 g

HARD-COOKED OR POACHED EGGS WITH SPINACH
Oeufs Durs ou Pochés Florentine aux Épinards

2 servings
PREPARATION TIME: 15 MIN

1½ pounds fresh spinach, trimmed
   and coarsely chopped or 10 oz
   package frozen spinach
1 small clove garlic, finely chopped
2 tbs water

pinch nutmeg
pepper, freshly ground
1 tbs any type vinegar
4 eggs

In a large skillet, combine spinach, garlic, and water. Cook over high heat 3–4 minutes until spinach is wilted and liquid evaporates. Season with nutmeg and pepper.

Meanwhile, boil water in a medium saucepan. Add vinegar. Break each egg into a cup then tip into simmering water. Poach eggs about 3 minutes or to desired doneness. (You may also hard cook the eggs in their shells. Add eggs to cold water; bring to a boil. Turn off heat; cover pan and let stand 10 minutes.)

Serve eggs on a bed of spinach.

CALORIES: 222   PROTEIN: 20 g

FLUFFY OMELET
Omelette Soufflée

2 servings
PREPARATION TIME: 15 MIN

2 egg yolks   *4 egg whites, at room temperature*
2 tbs lukewarm water   *2 tomatoes, quartered*
pepper, freshly ground   *2 sprigs parsley*

In a small bowl, beat egg yolks with lukewarm water and season with
pepper. In a mixer bowl, whip the egg whites until soft peaks form.
With a rubber spatula, gently mix the yolks into the whites. Pour the
mixture into a nonstick skillet, and cook over medium heat until the
bottom of the omelet is golden, about 3 minutes.

Place the skillet in the oven and brown the top. Decorate with the
tomatoes and parsley.

CALORIES: 134   PROTEIN: 13 g

Seafood

BROILED BASS WITH SEAWEED
Rôti de Bar au Varech

2 servings
PREPARATION TIME: 30 MIN

1 bunch watercress	*2 whole baby bass or trout (11 oz*
2 cups fresh sorrel	*each)*
3 egg whites	*½ oz Sevruga caviar (optional)*
pepper, freshly ground	

Preheat broiler.

Cut off long stems of watercress and remove the "ribs" of the sorrel.

Place the watercress and sorrel in a vegetable steamer, and steam over boiling water 3 minutes. Purée in blender or food processor.

In a mixer bowl, whip the egg whites until soft peaks form. Fold in the purée and season with pepper; pour into an oval gratin dish. Bake in 450 degree oven for 10 minutes until puffy and golden.

Meanwhile, broil the bass for about 10 minutes, turning once (5 minutes per side).

Sprinkle fish with Sevruga caviar just before serving.

Serve fish with the vegetable soufflé.

CALORIES: 332   PROTEIN: 44 g

GROUPER
WITH LIME AND COCONUT
St. Pierre au Citron Vert et au Coco

2 servings
PREPARATION TIME: 25–30 MIN

11 oz boned and cut-up grouper filets	¼ cup clam juice
¼ cup lime juice	¼ cup water
1 cup carrots, sliced	2 tsp unsweetened grated coconut
½ cup frozen peas	2 tbs plain low-fat yogurt
	1 tbs parsley, chopped

In a shallow glass baking dish, marinate grouper in lime juice for 15 minutes (or cover and refrigerate overnight).

Coat a large skillet with vegetable cooking spray; heat over high heat. Add fish and cook 3 minutes; turn and cook 3 minutes more.

Meanwhile, place carrots in vegetable steamer. Steam over boiling water for 5 minutes. Add peas and steam 2 minutes more.

Remove cooked fish from skillet. Add clam juice, water, and grated coconut; cook over high heat until liquid is reduced to about 2 tablespoons. Remove from heat and stir in yogurt.

Arrange fish on plates, top with sauce, and garnish with parsley.

CALORIES: 267   PROTEIN: 28 g

SALMON SCALLOPINI WITH FRESH VEGETABLES
Escalope de Saumon aux Primeurs

2 servings
PREPARATION TIME: 15 MIN

2 tsp olive oil
1 shallot, thinly sliced
1 cup eggplant, sliced
1 small zucchini, sliced
¼ cup green pepper, diced
2 fresh plum tomatoes, diced
1 clove garlic, pressed

pinch thyme
pepper, freshly ground
¼ cup water
11 oz salmon filets, cut in ¼-inch
   slices
parsley or chervil, chopped
lemon wedges

Heat 1 teaspoon of olive oil in a medium skillet. Add shallot and cook 1 minute over medium heat. Add eggplant; cover and cook 3 minutes. Add remaining vegetables, garlic, thyme, pepper, and water; cover and cook 3 minutes.

Meanwhile, heat remaining oil in a large skillet over medium high heat. Add salmon filets and cook 2 minutes on each side.

Serve salmon scallopini with vegetable stew. Sprinkle with chopped parsley and garnish with a lemon wedge.

CALORIES: 355   PROTEIN: 30 g

SALMON COOKED
AT LOW TEMPERATURE
Saumon Cuit à Basse Température

2 servings
PREPARATION TIME: 25 MIN

2 salmon filets, 6 oz each   *8 cherry tomatoes, split*
1½ cups green beans, trimmed

Preheat oven to 300 degrees.

Arrange salmon on a baking sheet. Bake 20 minutes.

After salmon has been cooking 10 minutes, place green beans in a vegetable steamer. Cover and steam over boiling water until almost tender, about 6 minutes. Add cherry tomatoes and steam 2 minutes more. Serve vegetables with the salmon.

CALORIES: 350   PROTEIN: 30 g

STEAMED MUSSELS
Moules Marinières

2 servings

PREPARATION TIME: 10 MIN

2 lb mussels
1 shallot, chopped

½ cup dry white wine
1 tbs parsley, chopped

Scrub the mussels; pull off the "beards."

Place the mussels in a large saucepan with the shallot and wine. Cover and cook over high heat 3–5 minutes, stirring once or twice. As soon as a mussel opens, remove it to serving plate. Continue cooking until all mussels are opened (or after 8 minutes, discard any mussels that have not opened).

Pour pan juices over mussels, and sprinkle with parsley.

CALORIES: 173   PROTEIN: 23 g

SCALLOPS GRATIN
WITH A FRINGE OF ENDIVE
Gratin de St. Jacques à l'Effiloché d'Endives

2 servings
PREPARATION TIME: 15 MIN

1 tsp butter or margarine
8 oz scallops
3 medium Belgian endives, trimmed
   and sliced

¼ cup dry white wine
1 whole clove
1 tbs light cream
pepper, freshly ground

Heat butter in a medium skillet over medium high heat. Add the scallops, and cook for 2 minutes, turning once.

Remove scallops and keep warm.

Add endive, wine, pepper, and clove to skillet; cover and cook 3 minutes. Remove from heat; stir in light cream.

With a slotted spoon, scoop half the endive on each plate. Arrange scallops on top, and spoon over any remaining juices.

CALORIES: 165   PROTEIN: 26 g

SEALED SCALLOPS
St. Jacques Lutées

2 servings
PREPARATION TIME: 20 MIN

1 tsp butter or margarine	*8 oz scallops*
¾ cup carrots, thinly sliced	*1 tsp chervil or parsley, chopped*
¼ cup green onions, sliced	*1 tbs clam broth mixed with*
1 cup mushrooms, sliced	*1 tbs dry white wine*

Preheat oven to 400 degrees.

Heat butter or margarine over medium high heat in a small skillet. Add carrots and cook 2 minutes. Add green onions and mushrooms and cook 3 minutes more.

Cut two 14-inch pieces of parchment or aluminum foil into circles or ovals. Fold each in half. Open and arrange scallops on one side of fold. Top with vegetable mixture. Sprinkle with chervil or parsley and spoon broth mixture over each.

Fold top half of paper down and fold two ends together, creasing at ½-inch intervals to completely enclose scallops. Bake 10 minutes. Split pouches with a sharp knife and serve.

CALORIES: 205   PROTEIN: 30 g

SCALLOPS À LA PROVENCE
Coquilles St. Jacques à la Provençale

2 servings
PREPARATION TIME: 15 MIN

8 oz large scallops, sliced into
* ½-inch rounds*
1 medium zucchini, thinly sliced

2 plum tomatoes, thinly sliced
1 tbs fresh basil, chopped
pepper, freshly ground

On two salad plates, arrange scallops, zucchini, and tomatoes alternately in a spiral pattern. Sprinkle with basil and pepper.

Cover each plate with plastic wrap and pierce plastic to vent. Microwave on high for 3 minutes, turning plates once halfway through cooking. Let stand covered 3 minutes before serving.

CALORIES: 140   PROTEIN: 27 g

SHRIMP PARFAITS
Parfait de Gambas

2 servings

PREPARATION TIME: 20 MIN

8 oz large raw shrimp, shelled and
   deveined
½ cup plain low-fat yogurt
2 tbs fresh basil, chopped
½ tsp lemon peel, grated

1 tsp lemon juice
⅛ tsp pepper, freshly ground
1 ½ cups romaine lettuce, shredded
1 tomato, chopped
2 basil leaves

Boil water in a medium saucepan. Add shrimp and cook 3 minutes. Rinse and drain shrimp; cool.

Combine yogurt, chopped basil, lemon peel, lemon juice, and pepper in a small bowl.

In two stemmed glasses, arrange one quarter of the lettuce. Top each with one quarter of the shrimp. Drizzle with some of the dressing and top with tomatoes. Repeat layering. Top each with a basil leaf.

CALORIES: 182

PROTEIN: 31 g

HODGEPODGE OF PINK SHRIMP
WITH OYSTERS

Méli-Mélo de Crevettes Roses aux Huîtres

2 servings
PREPARATION TIME: 10 MIN

*1 container (8 oz) fresh oysters,
    drained
4 oz shrimp, shelled and deveined
½ lemon
¼ cup plain low-fat yogurt*

*1 tsp fresh parsley, chopped
1 tsp fresh tarragon, chopped
1 tsp white horseradish
1 tsp lemon juice
lettuce leaves*

Bring a medium saucepan half full of water to a boil. Reduce heat and add oysters; simmer 2 minutes. Remove oysters with slotted spoon. Rinse and cool. Add shrimp to same water and cook 3 minutes; rinse and cool.

Peel lemon, discarding peel and white pith. Chop flesh into ¼-inch cubes.

Stir together yogurt, parsley, tarragon, and horseradish.

Line two plates with lettuce leaves. Arrange shrimp and oysters on lettuce. Sprinkle with cubed lemon and drizzle with the yogurt sauce.

Serve with a glass of white Burgundy (if permitted in plan).

CALORIES: 232   PROTEIN: 28 g

SHRIMP SALAD WITH SPROUTS

Cocktail de Crevettes au Soja

2 servings

PREPARATION TIME: 15–20 MIN

1 medium grapefruit
1 cup lamb's lettuce or bibb lettuce
½ cup artichoke hearts (canned or
frozen), sliced
4 oz shrimp, cooked, shelled,
deveined

½ cup plain low-fat yogurt
1 tsp Dijon mustard
2 tsp catsup
3 drops Tabasco
1 cup bean sprouts

Using a sharp knife, remove the skin and white pith of the grapefruit; cut into sections.

Arrange lettuce in centers of two plates. Surround with artichoke slices, grapefruit sections, and shrimp. Blend together yogurt, Dijon mustard, catsup, and Tabasco. Drizzle over salad. Top each salad with bean sprouts.

CALORIES: 153

PROTEIN: 20 g

RED MULLET OR SNAPPER
WITH FRESH FENNEL
Petit Rouget au Fenouil Frais

2 servings
PREPARATION TIME: 15 MIN

1 small bulb fennel, cored and thinly
   sliced
½ cup water
2 tbs light cream
11 oz red mullet or red snapper filet

pepper to taste
¼ tsp fresh thyme
2 tsp salmon caviar
1 tsp chervil or parsley, chopped

Preheat broiler.

Arrange the fennel slices in a medium skillet; add water. Cover
and cook over high heat until fennel is tender, about 6 minutes.
Drain fennel; return to skillet and add cream. Cook until heated
through.

Meanwhile, season the mullet or snapper filets with pepper and
thyme. Broil 3 inches from heat source, until opaque throughout,
5–6 minutes.

Arrange fish on plates; top with salmon caviar and chopped chervil; serve with fennel.

CALORIES: 323   PROTEIN: 35 g

FILET OF SOLE
WITH CUCUMBER PURÉE
Filet de Sole à la Purée de Concombre

2 servings
PREPARATION TIME: 25 MIN

½ small bulb fennel, sliced
1 shallot, chopped
2 filets of a large sole
½ cup clam juice
2 tbs sauternes or other sweet white
    wine

1 medium cucumber, peeled and
    seeded
pepper, freshly ground

Preheat oven to 450 degrees.

Place fennel in vegetable steamer and steam over boiling water 6–8 minutes, until tender.

Meanwhile, place shallots in bottom of a shallow baking dish; arrange sole filets on top. Pour the clam juice and sauternes on top. Cover and bake 8 minutes.

While the fish is baking, purée the cucumber in a blender or food processor. Transfer to a small saucepan and heat through. Season with pepper.

Serve the sole filets topped with cucumber purée and fennel.

CALORIES: 213   PROTEIN: 30 g

SOLE WITH GRAPES
Sole aux Raisins

2 servings
PREPARATION TIME: 15 MIN

2 filets of sole (11 oz)
6 romaine lettuce leaves
pepper, freshly ground
¾ cup green seedless grapes, cut in
* half (set aside 8 pieces for*
* garnish)*

⅓ cup water
1 tbs lemon juice

Preheat broiler. Line broiler pan with aluminum foil. Arrange the sole filets on two lettuce leaves. Place on broiler pan. Season with pepper.

In a small skillet, combine grapes, water, and lemon juice; bring to a boil. Cook until liquid is reduced to about 2 tablespoons.

Broil sole 3 inches from heat source for 5 minutes.

Meanwhile, finely shred remaining lettuce. Arrange the lettuce on two plates. Top with a fish filet. Pour any juices from fish into skillet with grapes; boil 1 minute, then spoon over fish. Garnish with reserved grapes.

CALORIES: 173   PROTEIN: 28 g

TROUT FILETS
WITH SMALL VEGETABLES
Filets de Truite aux Petits Légumes

2 servings

PREPARATION TIME: 15 MIN

1 shallot, thinly sliced

1 small zucchini, cut in 1/3-inch cubes

1/2 cup artichoke hearts (frozen or canned), sliced

1/4 cup green pepper, diced

1 plum tomato, diced

1 clove garlic, pressed

1 tbs fresh dill, chopped

1/4 cup water

1 tsp olive oil

12 oz trout filets

lemon wedge

Brown the shallot in a small nonstick skillet over medium high heat. Add remaining vegetables, garlic, dill, and water; cover and cook for 5 minutes.

Meanwhile, heat oil in a medium skillet over medium high heat. Add trout filets and cook 2 minutes. Turn and cook 2–3 minutes more. Serve trout with vegetables. Garnish with a lemon wedge.

CALORIES: 235   PROTEIN: 31 g

TROUT IN SALT
Truite au Sel

2 servings
PREPARATION TIME: 30 MIN

1 large trout for two persons (18 oz
   to 22 oz)
2 sprigs parsley
1 sprig dill
2 sprigs chervil

1 box kosher salt
4 leeks, sliced
½ cup water
1 tsp butter or margarine

Preheat oven to 475 degrees. Line a large baking sheet with aluminum foil.

Stuff cavity of fish with the herbs.

Pour a ½-inch layer of salt on to foil. Arrange fish on top. Cover entirely with rest of salt. Bake for 20 minutes.

After the fish has been baking about 10 minutes, place the leeks in a medium saucepan with water and butter or margarine.

Cover and heat to boiling; reduce heat and simmer until leeks are tender, about 10 minutes.

Serve the salt shell on a dish; break and take the trout out. Serve leeks on the side.

CALORIES: 240   PROTEIN: 30 g

STEAMED BABY LOBSTER WITH VEGETABLES
Petit Homard à la Vapeur

2 servings
PREPARATION TIME: 20 MIN

¾ cup water
½ cup clam juice
¼ tsp thyme
1 cup leeks, sliced

2 small lobsters (about 1 lb each)
1 cup cauliflower
1 cup carrots, sliced

In a pot large enough to hold lobsters, bring water and clam juice to a boil with thyme. Add leeks and lobsters; cover and steam 7 minutes. Add cauliflower and carrots, and steam 5 minutes more.

Serve lobsters with the steamed vegetables.

CALORIES: 182   PROTEIN: 30 g

MEDALLIONS OF LOBSTER SCENTED WITH WILD HERBS

Médaillons de Langoustes aux Vapeurs d'Herbes Sauvages

2 servings

PREPARATION TIME: 35 MIN

1 cup water	1 whole clove
½ cup clam juice	¼ tsp black peppercorns
¼ cup dry white wine	1 stalk celery, sliced
2 sprigs chervil	1 sprig fresh coriander
2 bay leaves	1 clove garlic, unpeeled
2 twigs thyme	8 oz lobster meat, sliced
1 carrot, peeled and sliced	1 tbs light cream

In a medium saucepan, combine water, clam juice, wine, chervil, bay leaves, thyme, carrot, clove, peppercorns, celery, coriander, and garlic clove; heat to boiling. Boil 10 minutes. Strain broth. Return broth to saucepan and reduce heat to a simmer. Add lobster meat and simmer 2 minutes.

Remove from heat and stir in cream. Spoon into soup bowls and serve.

CALORIES: 220   PROTEIN: 31 g

MIXED GRILLED FISH

Arlequin de Poissons Grillés

2 servings

PREPARATION TIME: 20 MIN

10 oz fresh spinach, trimmed and
    rinsed
2 tbs water
4 oz turbot filet

4 oz bass filet
1 large scallop, halved horizontally
2 jumbo shrimp, peeled and deveined
1 tbs light cream

Preheat grill or broiler.

Place the spinach in a large skillet with water. Cover and cook 3 minutes; uncover and cook until water evaporates.

Arrange all fish on broiler rack. Broil 3 inches from heat source until fish is just opaque and shrimp is pink, 3–4 minutes.

Stir cream into spinach and heat. Divide fish and spinach between two plates and serve.

CALORIES: 308   PROTEIN: 42 g

MIXED SEAFOOD FLAVORED
WITH WILD HERBS
Petite Nage aux Senteurs d'Herbe Folle

2 servings
PREPARATION TIME: 25 MIN

¼ cup clam juice
½ cup sauternes or other sweet
  white wine
¾ cup carrots, thinly sliced
½ cup leeks, thinly sliced
½ cup celery, thinly sliced

5 oz John Dory filet, boned and
  skinned
5 oz salmon filet, boned and skinned
1 large scallop, halved horizontally
2 jumbo shrimp, peeled and deveined
4 sprigs chervil or fennel

In a medium saucepan, bring the clam juice and wine to a boil. Add the carrots, leeks, and celery; cover and simmer 5 minutes. Add the John Dory and salmon; simmer 3–5 minutes. Add the scallop and shrimp; simmer 2 minutes.

Serve the fish in a soup plate with the vegetables and the broth.

CALORIES: 333   PROTEIN: 37 g

FISH STEW WITH HERBS
Pot-au-Feu de la Mer

2 servings
PREPARATION TIME: 20 MIN

4 cups water
¼ cup white wine or cider vinegar
1 onion, sliced
½ cup carrots, sliced
½ cup celery, sliced
1 whole clove

1 tbs parsley, chopped
½ tsp fresh thyme
1 bay leaf
⅛ tsp pepper, coarsely ground
1 to 1¼ lb whole fish or 12 oz fish
   filets

In a saucepan large enough to hold the fish, combine water, wine or vinegar, onion, carrots, celery, clove, parsley, thyme, and pepper. Boil for 15 minutes. Reduce heat to medium. Add fish and simmer until done. A whole fish will take 10–15 minutes. Filets will cook in 5 minutes.

Serve fish in bowls with vegetables and broth.

CALORIES: 145   PROTEIN: 27 g

Desserts

BAKED APPLE SURPRISE
Pommes Surprises au Four

2 servings
PREPARATION TIME: 15 MIN

2 golden delicious apples   *1 packet artificial sweetener*
1 egg white   *½ cup unsweetened applesauce*

Preheat oven to 400 degrees.

Core each apple without cutting through bottom; hollow out to form a wide cavity. Place apples in a shallow baking dish.

In a mixer bowl, whip egg whites until soft peaks form. Fold in artificial sweetener and applesauce. Scoop into apples. Bake 12–15 minutes until filling is puffy and golden.

CALORIES: 138   PROTEIN: 2 g

BAKED ORANGE
Orange au Four

2 servings
PREPARATION TIME: 10 MIN

2 oranges   *pinch cinnamon*
1 egg white

Preheat oven to 450 degrees.

Using a small sharp knife, remove all peel and white pith from the oranges. Quarter each orange and arrange in two oven-proof dishes.

In a small mixer bowl, whip egg white until soft peaks form. Scoop half the egg white onto each orange. Bake 10 minutes or until meringue is browned. Sprinkle with cinnamon and serve.

CALORIES: 67   PROTEIN: 3 g

CINNAMON-FLAVORED STRAWBERRIES
Gratin de Fraises à la Cannelle

2 servings
PREPARATION TIME: 20 MIN

1 cup strawberries, hulled and
    quartered
2 egg whites

2 packets artificial sweetener
½ tsp cinnamon

Preheat oven to 450 degrees.

Arrange strawberries in a small gratin dish or two 1-cup soufflé dishes.

In a mixer bowl, whip the egg whites to soft peaks. Beat in the artificial sweetener and cinnamon.

Pour over strawberries and bake until golden and puffed, about 10 minutes. Serve at once.

CALORIES: 38   PROTEIN: 4 g

STRAWBERRIES IN CHAMPAGNE
Soupe de Fraises au Champagne

2 servings
PREPARATION TIME: 10 MIN

1½ cups strawberries, hulled and
    quartered
1 packet artificial sweetener

¾ cup champagne (or other
    sparkling wine)
1 tbs fresh mint, chopped

Combine the strawberries and artificial sweetener in a bowl. Place the strawberries in two soup plates; add the champagne and sprinkle with the mint.

CALORIES: 86   PROTEIN: 1 g

FROZEN YOGURT
WITH KIWI SAUCE
Yogourt Glacé au Coulis de Kiwi

2 servings
PREPARATION TIME: 5 MIN PLUS FREEZING

¾ cup plain low-fat yogurt
2 packets artificial sweetener
½ tsp vanilla extract

1 kiwi fruit, peeled
1 tsp lemon juice

In a bowl, stir together yogurt, artificial sweetener, and vanilla. Pour into two ½-cup ramekins; cover and freeze 45 minutes.

In a blender, purée kiwi with lemon juice.

Spoon the kiwi purée onto two dessert dishes. Unmold the frozen yogurts onto the purée (dipping the molds briefly in hot water to loosen, if necessary) and serve.

CALORIES: 70   PROTEIN: 5 g

KIWI PETALS
WITH STRAWBERRY PURÉE
Pétales de Kiwi au Jus de Fraises

2 servings
PREPARATION TIME: 5 MIN

1 cup strawberries, hulled and
  quartered

1 tsp lemon juice
2 kiwi fruits, peeled and thinly sliced

In a blender, purée the strawberries and the lemon juice. Pour the strawberry purée onto two dessert plates. Decorate with a rosette of kiwis.

CALORIES: 50   PROTEIN: 1 g

TWO-FRUIT MOUSSE
Mousse aux Deux Fruits

2 servings
PREPARATION TIME: 10 MIN PLUS REFRIGERATION

¼ cup lemon juice
1 packet gelatin
½ cup orange juice
1 tsp orange peel, grated

½ tsp lemon peel, grated
¾ cup plain low-fat yogurt
2 egg whites
2 packets artificial sweetener

Pour lemon juice into a small saucepan; sprinkle with a small amount of the gelatin. Set aside for 5 minutes.

In a large bowl, whisk together orange juice and orange and lemon peels. Heat gelatin in pan of water over low heat to dissolve. Stir into orange juice mixture. Whisk in yogurt.

In mixer bowl, whip egg whites until soft peaks form; beat in artificial sweetener. Fold whites into orange mixture.

Pour into 1-cup ramekins; cover and refrigerate for 3 hours.

CALORIES: 98   PROTEIN: 9 g

FRESH FRUIT ASPIC WITH EXOTIC FLAVORS

Aspic de Fruits Frais aux Saveurs Exotiques

2 servings
PREPARATION TIME: 10 MIN PLUS REFRIGERATION

½ cup plus 2 tbs water
1 tsp gelatin
1 cup fresh fruits, sliced

1 mint teabag
½ packet artificial sweetener

Place 2 tbs water in a small saucepan. Sprinkle with the gelatin. In teacup, steep tea in ½ cup boiled water for 3 minutes; remove teabag.

Meanwhile, arrange fruit in two 5-ounce custard cups. Heat gelatin over low heat until melted. Remove from heat; add tea and artificial sweetener. Pour evenly over fruit. Cover and refrigerate at least 1 hour or up to 24 hours.

CALORIES: 76   PROTEIN: 1 g

FRUIT SKEWERS
Brochettes de Fruits en Papillotes

2 servings

PREPARATION TIME: 15 MIN

1 cup strawberries, hulled	½ cup pineapple, diced
1 kiwi fruit, peeled and cut in	2 tbs fresh mint, chopped
¾-inch cubes	1 tsp vanilla extract

Combine all ingredients in a bowl. Arrange fruit on wooden skewers, alternating strawberries, kiwi, and pineapple. Serve chilled.

These may also be baked en papillote. Preheat oven to 400 degrees. Arrange skewers on half a sheet of aluminum foil. Fold other half over and crimp edges to seal. Bake 10 minutes.

CALORIES: 64   PROTEIN: 1 g

LOW-CALORIE DARK CHOCOLATE MOUSSE
Mousse au Chocolat Noir Allégé

2 servings

PREPARATION TIME: 5 MIN PLUS FREEZING

2 egg whites	1 oz unsweetened chocolate, melted
2 packets artificial sweetener	

In mixer bowl, whip egg whites until soft peaks form. Beat in artificial sweetener. Gently fold in chocolate.

Fill two 1-cup ramekins; freeze for 2 hours.

CALORIES: 88   PROTEIN: 5 g

Appendix

The Recommended Dietary Allowances (RDA)

These are the nutrients your body needs on a daily basis; any vitamin and mineral supplements you take should contain approximately the same amounts.

Age (years)	Weight (kg)	Weight (lbs)	Height (cm)	Height (in)	Protein (g)	Vitamin A (RE)[2]	Vitamin D (mcg)[3]	Vitamin E (mg)	Vitamin C (mg)	Thiamine (mg)
Infants										
0.0–0.5	6	13	60	24	kg × 2.2	420	10	3	35	0.3
0.5–1.0	9	20	71	28	kg × 2.0	400	10	4	35	0.5
Children										
1–3	13	29	90	35	23	400	10	5	45	0.7
4–6	20	44	112	44	30	500	10	6	45	0.9
7–10	28	62	132	52	34	700	10	7	45	1.2
Males										
11–14	45	99	157	62	45	1,000	10	8	50	1.4
15–18	66	145	176	69	56	1,000	10	10	60	1.4
19–22	70	154	177	70	56	1,000	7.5	10	60	1.5
23–50	70	154	178	70	56	1,000	5	10	60	1.4
51 +	70	154	178	70	56	1,000	5	10	60	1.2
Females										
11–14	46	101	157	62	46	800	10	8	50	1.1
15–18	55	120	163	64	46	800	10	8	60	1.1
19–22	55	120	163	64	44	800	7.5	8	60	1.1
23–50	55	120	163	64	44	800	5	8	60	1.0
51 +	55	120	163	64	44	800	5	8	60	1.0
Pregnant[1]					+ 30	+ 200	+ 5	+ 2	+ 20	+ 0.4
Lactating[1]					+ 20	+ 400	+ 5	+ 3	+ 40	+ 0.5

[1] Pregnant and lactating women are well advised to take iron supplements as recommended by their physician.

[2] 1 RE = 5 IU.

[3] 1 mcg = 40 IU.

[4] One mg equivalent is equal to 1 mg of niacin or 60 mg of tryptophan (tryptophan can be converted to niacin by the body).

Reproduced from Recommended Dietary Allowances, 9th ed. (1980), National Academy of Sciences, Washington, D.C.

Ribo-flavin (mg)	Niacin[4] (mg equiv.)	Vitamin B6 (mg)	Folacin (mcg)	Vitamin B12 (mcg)	Calcium (mg)	Phos-phorus (mg)	Mag-nesium (mg)	Iron (mg)	Zinc (mg)	Iodine (mcg)
0.4	6	0.3	30	0.5	360	240	50	10	3	40
0.6	8	0.6	45	1.5	540	360	70	15	5	50
0.8	9	0.9	100	2.0	800	800	150	15	10	70
1.0	11	1.3	200	2.5	800	800	200	10	10	90
1.4	16	1.6	300	3.0	800	800	250	10	10	120
1.6	18	1.8	400	3.0	1,200	1,200	350	18	15	150
1.7	18	2.0	400	3.0	1,200	1,200	400	18	15	150
1.7	19	2.2	400	3.0	800	800	350	10	15	150
1.6	18	2.2	400	3.0	800	800	350	10	15	150
1.4	16	2.2	400	3.0	800	800	350	10	15	150
1.3	15	1.8	400	3.0	1,200	1,200	300	18	15	150
1.3	14	2.0	400	3.0	1,200	1,200	300	18	15	150
1.3	14	2.0	400	3.0	800	800	300	18	15	150
1.2	13	2.0	400	3.0	800	800	300	18	15	150
1.2	13	2.0	400	3.0	800	800	300	10	15	150
+0.3	+2	+0.6	+400	+1.0	+400	+400	+150		+5	+25
+0.5	+5	+0.5	+100	+1.0	+400	+400	+150		+10	+50

About the Authors

PAUL SACHET, M.D., has been a nutrition consultant in the world-famous nutrition department of the Bichat Hospital in Paris for more than ten years. A specialist in eating disorders, obesity and lipid metabolism, he is the author of numerous articles and books in his field and has chaired conferences in France and abroad. In addition, he was the scientific organizer of four international meetings on nutrition in Paris.

Dr. Sachet is a recipient of the prestigious French Academy of Medicine Award and a member of numerous learned societies. He is married and has three children.

BRIAN L. G. MORGAN, Ph.D., formerly of Columbia University's Institute of Human Nutrition, is one of the world's foremost educators, writers, and researchers in the field of human nutrition. He has counseled many people with weight problems and has written numerous books and articles dealing with nutrition and health, including *Nutrition Prescription, Brain Food,* and *The Food and Drug Interaction Guide.*

ROBERTA MORGAN is a leading health and nutrition writer, with eleven published books to her credit and numerous magazine articles for such publications as *Self, American Health,* and *Family Circle.* Her books include *Brain Food, The Emotional Pharmacy,* and *Hormones.* She has also published several newsletters in the field of nutrition, including *Food and Fitness,* and *Nutrition and Health* (from Columbia University's Institute of Human Nutrition).